Instructor's Manual
to
Accompany

Diversified Health Occupations 7th EDITION

Louise Simmers, MEd, RN

Karen Simmers-Nartker, BSN, RN

Sharon Simmers-Kobelak, BBA

DELMAR
CENGAGE Learning™

Australia Canada Mexico Singapore Spain United Kingdom United States

DELMAR
CENGAGE Learning™

Instructor's Manual to accompany Diversified Health Occupations
7th Edition
by Louise Simmers, MEd, RN,
Karen Simmers-Nartker, BSN, RN, and
Sharon Simmers-Kobelak, BBA

Vice President, Career and Professional Editorial: Dave Garza

Director of Learning Solutions: Matthew Kane

Managing Editor: Marah Bellegarde

Acquisitions Editor: Matthew Seeley

Senior Product Manager: Juliet Steiner

Editorial Assistant: Megan Tarquinio

Vice President, Marketing Career and Professional: Jennifer McAvey

Marketing Manager: Michele McTighe

Marketing Coordinator: Vanessa Carlson

Technology Product Manager: Mary Colleen Liburdi

Technology Project Manager: Benjamin Knapp

Production Director: Carolyn Miller

Senior Art Director: Jack Pendleton

Content Product Manager: Anne Sherman

Library of Congress Control Number: 2007941692

2007941692

ISBN-13: 978-1-4180-3025-4
ISBN-10: 1-4180-3025-2

Delmar Cengage Learning
5 Maxwell Drive
Clifton Park, NY 12065-2919
USA

Cengage Learning is a leading provider of customized learning solutions with office locations around the globe, including Singapore, the United Kingdom, Australia, Mexico, Brazil, and Japan. Locate your local office at:

international.cengage.com/region

Cengage Learning products are represented in Canada by Nelson Education, Ltd.

For your lifelong learning solutions, visit **delmar.cengage.com**

Visit our corporate website at **cengage.com**

NOTICE TO THE READER
Publisher does not warrant or guarantee any of the products described herein or perform any independent analysis in connection with any of the product information contained herein. Publisher does not assume, and expressly disclaims, any obligation to obtain and include information other than that provided to it by the manufacturer. The reader is expressly warned to consider and adopt all safety precautions that might be indicated by the activities herein and to avoid all potential hazards. By following the instructions contained herein, the reader willingly assumes all risks in connection with such instructions. The publisher makes no representation or warranties of any kind, including but not limited to, the warranties of fitness for particular purpose or merchantability, nor are any such representations implied with respect to the material set forth herein, and the publisher takes no responsibility with respect to such material. The publisher shall not be liable for any special, consequential, or exemplary damages resulting, in whole or part, from the readers' use of, or reliance upon, this material.

Printed in the U.S.A.
3 4 5 6 7 XXX 12 11 10

CONTENTS

Preface

The text and workbook for *Diversified Health Occupations,* 7th edition, were designed to provide the beginning health science technology education (HSTE) student with the basic knowledge and entry-level skills required for a wide variety of health occupations.

- The material will not replace the instructor, who is still an important element for student success. However, by using the material correctly, students can work more independently and master many skills at beginning levels of achievement. Students know what is expected of them as definite standards are set. Evaluations are objective, and quality of performance is stressed. In this *Instructor's Manual,* suggested answers for the assignment sheets in the workbook are given.
- Because regulations vary from state to state regarding procedures that can be performed by health science technology education (HSTE) students, it is important for the instructor to check specific state regulations. Stressing legal responsibilities to students is an important function of any HSTE instructor.
- Always remember that a HSTE instructor is providing a valuable service. The material in the text and workbook has been prepared to make the job a little easier. One hopes it will help many students become competent health care workers.
- A *Teacher's Resource Kit* to accompany *Diversified Health Occupations,* 7th edition, is available for purchase. This kit provides a complete guide to implementing a Diversified Health Occupations course. The kit contains instructional strategies and explains how to apply content to applied academics and the National Health Care Skill Standards. It also provides classroom management ideas, lesson plans, tests, classroom activities, leadership development activities, suggestions for Internet searches, transparency masters, and lists of additional resources.
- An Electronic Classroom Manager to Accompany *Diversified Health Occupations* 7th Edition is also available from the publisher. It contains a *Computerized Test Bank* of over 1,800 questions that can be used to create quizzes and tests, an electronic version of this *Instructor's Manual,* a *PowerPoint® Presentation* with approximately 1,000 slides for use in classroom instruction, an *Image Library* with electronic versions of all of the transparency masters for use in giving electronic presentations and creating customized assignments and worksheets, and an Animations Library with 17 multimedia animations providing narration and explanation of difficult to visualize anatomical and physiological processes for use in classroom presentations.

Available for *Diversified Health Occupations,* 7th edition:
- Teacher's Resource Kit: 1-4180-3023-6
- Workbook: 1-4180-3022-8
- Electronic Classroom Manager: 1-4180-3024-4
- WebTutor™: WebCT® version: 1-4180-3026-0
- WebTutor™: Blackboard® version: 1-4180-3027-9
- Online Companion: 1-4180-3028-7

CHAPTER 1 HISTORY AND TRENDS OF HEALTH CARE

A. Matching

1. C	6. U	11. A	16. R
2. Q	7. M	12. G	17. P
3. N	8. I	13. S	18. H
4. L	9. D	14. B	19. W
5. V	10. E	15. O	20. T

B. Completion and Short Answer

1. evil spirits and demons
2. good diet, fresh air, cleanliness, exercise
3. prayer and divine intervention
4. (any 4 of the following) bubonic plague, smallpox, diphtheria, tuberculosis, typhoid, malaria
5. allowed doctors to view body organs and see the connections between different systems; provided a better understanding of anatomy and physiology
6. allowed physicians to see organisms to small to be seen by the human eye; provided the first observation of pathogenic organisms
7. plants and herbs
8. allowed physicians to listen to internal body sounds
9. (any 4 of the following) Florence Nightingale: began formal training for nurses; Elizabeth Blackwell: first female physician in the United States; Dorthea Dix: Superintendent of Female Nurses of the Army; Elizabeth Garrett Anderson: first female physician in Britain; Clara Barton: founded the American Red Cross; Lillian Wald: established the Henry Street Settlement
10. began the search for gene therapy to cure inherited diseases
11. computer technology
12. answers will be individualized; make sure students have explained why they want the advancement
13. a. cost containment: trying to control the rising cost of health care, keeping health care at levels individuals can afford
    b. diagnostic related groups (DRGs): certain diagnoses classified in one payment group, done to control rising costs, leads to early release from hospitals and need for other facilities
    c. energy conservation: monitoring the use of energy to control costs and conserve resources
    d. home health care: providing care in the home, increasing because of early hospital release resulting from DRGs, desire of patients for care in home
    e. geriatric care: care of the elderly, increasing because of increase in life span and large number of people who are approaching this age group
    f. telemedicine: use of video, audio, and computer systems to provide medical and/or health care services
    g. wellness: state of being in optimum health, more awareness of good health and more stress on preventing or delaying disease
    h. alternative and complementary methods of health care: individuals seek other types of treatment for a variety of conditions, health care worker must respect person's right to receive this care
14. (Any 4 of the following) complete a state-approved training program, pass a written and/or competency examination, continuing education, periodic evaluation of performance, retraining and/or retesting if the assistant does not work in a health care facility for more than two years
15. care that promotes physical, emotional, social, intellectual, and spiritual well-being
16. complementary therapies are used in conjunction with conventional medical therapies; alternative therapies are used in place of conventional medical therapies
17. each person is unique and may require different medical treatments and a variety of CAM therapies
18. answers will be individualized; make sure students have included reasons why a national health care plan should or should not be established

CHAPTER 2 HEALTH CARE SYSTEMS

1. a. laboratory, b. health maintenance, c. long-term care, d. industrial health, e. emergency care, f. mental health, g. clinic, h. rehabilitation, i. hospital
2. a. long-term care facilities, b. emergency care services, c. mental health facilities, d. industrial health care centers, e. dental offices, f. laboratories, g. home health care agencies, h. rehabilitation facilities, i. genetic counseling facilities
3. private or proprietary, religious, nonprofit or voluntary, government
4. residential care facilities: provide basic physical and emotional care

   extended care facilities: provide skilled nursing and rehabilitative care

   independent living facilities: provide assistance with meals, housekeeping, laundry, transportation, and basic medical care to individuals who can care for themselves
5. (Any 3 of the following) diagnosis, treatment, examinations, basic laboratory tests, minor surgery
6. (Any 3 of the following) group of doctors who share a facility, surgical clinics, urgent care clinics, rehabilitation clinics, specialty clinics, outpatient clinics, health department clinics, medical center clinics
7. (Any 3 of the following) nursing care, personal care, therapy, homemaking
8. care that provides support and comfort to allow a person to die with dignity
9. help patient with physical or mental disabilities obtain maximum self-care and function
10. (Any 3 of the following) provide emergency care for accidents or sudden illness, perform tests for health conditions, promote health education, maintain safe and sanitary environment
11. World Health Organization, U.S. Department of Health and Human Services, National Institutes of Health, Occupational Safety and Health Administration, Agency for Health Care Policy and Research
12. (Any 4 of the following) immunization for disease control, inspections for environmental health and sanitation, communicable disease control, collection of statistics and records, health education, clinics
13. a. donations, membership fees, fund-raisers, federal or state grants, b. (Any 2 of the following) study disease, provide funding for research, promote public education, provide special services to victims of disease, provide treatment centers, supply information about other community agencies
14. a. premium: payment made to insurance company
    b. deductible: amount that must be paid by the patient for needed services before the policy begins to pay
    c. 75/25% coinsurance: company pays 75% and patient pays 25% of expense
    d. copayment: specific amount of money a patient pays for a particular service
    e. HMOs: Health Maintenance Organizations
    f. PPOs: Preferred Provider Organizations
15. a. (Any of the following) monthly fee the same regardless of the amount of care, care directed toward preventive care, ready access to health examinations and early treatment
    b. required to use only HMO-affiliated health care providers
16. use a PPO that requires that specific hospitals or doctors be used
17. Medicare: almost all individuals over 65, any person with a disability who has had Social Security benefits for at least two years, any person with end-stage renal disease

    Medicaid: individuals with low incomes, children who qualify for public assistance, individuals who are physically disabled or blind

    State Children's Health Insurance Program: uninsured children of working families who earn too little to afford private insurance but too much to be eligibal for Medicaid

    TRICARE: all active duty military personnel and their families, survivors of military personnel, retired members of the armed forces

    Workers' Compensation: workers who are injured on the job
18. developed because of rising cost of health care; principle is that all health care provided must have a purpose
19. Health Insurance Portability and Accountability Act (HIPAA)
20. shows a line of authority to indicate areas of responsibility and leads to efficient operation

CHAPTER 3 CAREERS IN HEALTH CARE

A. Matching

1. T	6. K	11. J	16. U	21. C
2. E	7. B	12. A	17. H	22. M
3. F	8. W	13. L	18. Q	23. O
4. I	9. S	14. D	19. R	24. X
5. P	10. V	15. N	20. G	

B. Health Careers Search

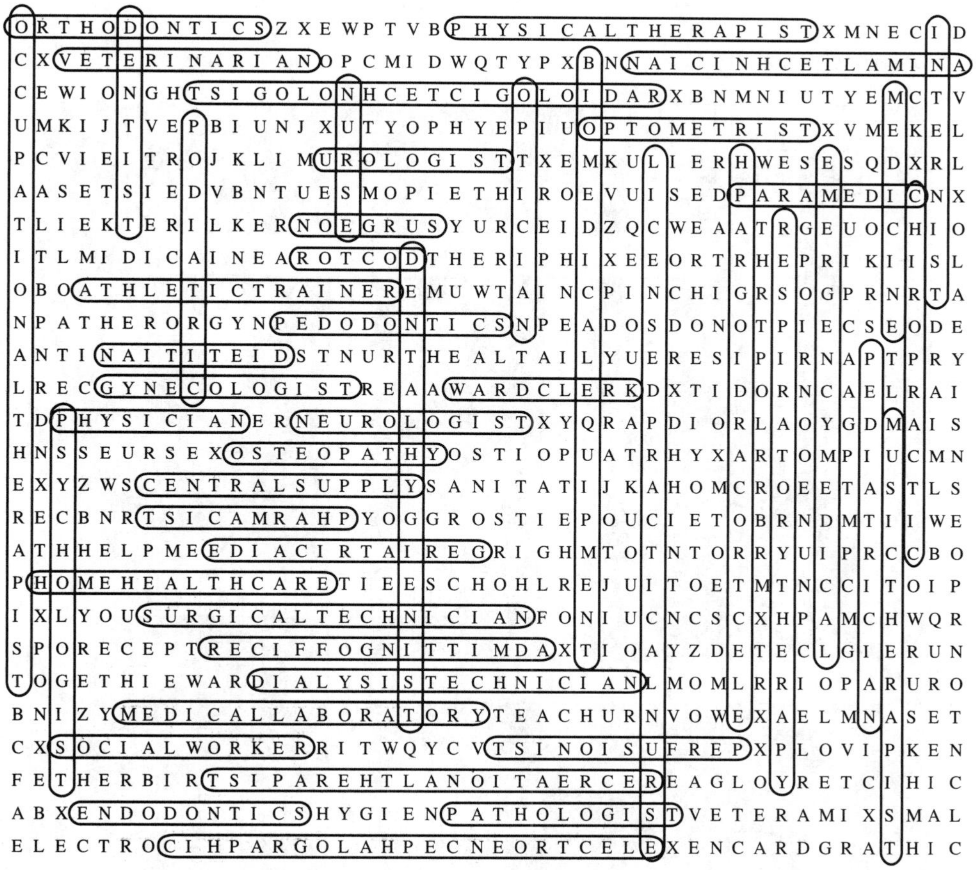

C. Completion and Short Answer

1. Associate: complete a two-year course of study at community college or vocational-technical school
   Bachelor's: usually four-year course of study at college or university
   Master's: usually one or more years of study beyond a bachelor's degree
2. a. certification, b. licensure, c. registration
3. obtain additional hours of education in a specific health care career to renew a license or maintain a certificate
4. technician usually requires two-year associate degree or three to four years of on-the-job training or special health occupations education; technologist usually requires at least three to four years of college in addition to work experience, usually bachelor's and, at times, master's degree
5. workers who can perform in a variety of occupations; because of high cost of health care, smaller facilities or rural areas cannot afford to hire a specialist for every aspect of care
6. individual who organizes, manages, and assumes the risk of a business
   (Any 3 of the following) well motivated, self-confident, responsible, creative, independent
7. a. orthodontics, b. ophthalmologist, c. psychiatrist, d. oral surgeon, e. neurologist, f. gynecologist, g. urologist, h. family physician, i. periodontics, j. oncologist, k. cardiologist, l. gerontologist, m. pediatrician, n. obstetrician

8. a. dental hygienist, b. electroencephalographic technologist, c. radiologic technologist, d. emergency medical technician, e. health information (medical records) technician, f. health care administrator, g. geriatric assistant, h. pharmacist, i. recreational therapist, j. optometrist, k. embalmer, l. epidemiologist, m. forensic science technician, n. medical interpreter/translator, o. genetic counselor, p. process technician
9. answers will be individualized; make sure students include the duties of the careers, the educational requirements, and a brief explanation of why the careers were chosen
10. check letters for correct form, spelling, punctuation, and so on

CHAPTER 4 PERSONAL AND PROFESSIONAL QUALITIES OF A HEALTH CARE WORKER

A. Answers to crossword puzzle

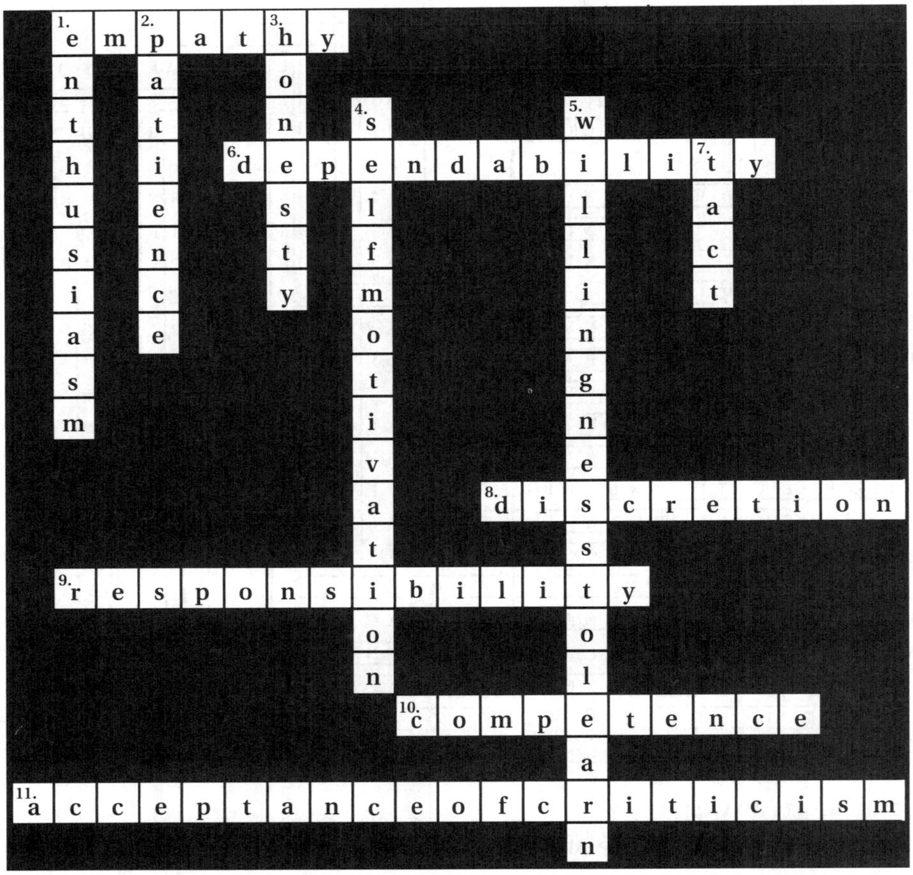

B. Characteristic Profile: Answers will be individualized; make sure students have defined at least eight (8) different characteristics in the description.

C. Completion and Short Answer

1. diet: provides body with materials for optimum health
   rest: provides energy and ability to deal with stress
   exercise: maintains circulation; improves muscle tone, enhances mental attitude, aids in weight control, and contributes to more restful sleep
   good posture: prevents fatigue and puts less stress on muscles
   avoid use of tobacco and drugs: prevents damage to body systems
2. (Any 3 of the following) neat, well-fitting, clean, free from wrinkles, white or neutral undergarments
3. follow standards established by place of employment
4. (Any 3 of the following) fit well, provide good support, have low heels, avoid sandals or open-toe shoes, clean daily, clean/replace shoelaces frequently
5. (Any 3 of the following) daily bath or shower, use of deodorant or antiperspirant, good oral hygiene, clean undergarments

6. avoid injuring patients, avoid transmitting germs, prevent torn or punctured gloves
7. hand cream or lotion
8. keep hair from touching patient, falling on a tray/equipment, or blocking necessary vision
9. watch; wedding ring; small, pierced earrings
10. can interfere with patient care and detract from professional appearance
11. create a natural appearance and add to a person's attractiveness
12. detract from a professional appearance, are prohibited in many health care facilities
13. (Any 4 of the following) message must be clear, sender delivers message effectively, receiver must hear or receive message, receiver must understand message, avoid interruptions or distractions
14. a. not in terms patient can understand
    b. receiver may not be able to hear message
    c. distraction of radio interferes with message
    d. using slang or incorrect grammar
    e. shows lack of interest
    f. poor listening
15. paying attention to and making an effort to hear what the other person is saying
16. lets speaker know statements are being heard and allows speaker to clarify a message
17. facial expressions, body language, gestures, eye contact, touch
18. often conveys a message that is different from the verbal communication
19. physical disabilities, psychological attitudes and prejudice, cultural diversity
20. (Any 4 of the following) use soft tone of voice, describe events, announce your presence, explain sounds or noises, use touch when appropriate
21. (any 4 of the following) allow patient to express fear, encourage patient to talk about feelings, avoid arguing, remain calm, talk in a soft and nonthreatening tone of voice, provide quality care
22. values, beliefs, attitudes, and customs shared by a group of people and passed from one generation to the next
23. individual answers should include:
    a. check with immediate supervisor because patient may be allowed to leave article in place
    b. allow patient to express this belief and encourage patient to talk, do not preach your own religion
    c. continue with communication; patient may not feel comfortable with eye contact but still may be listening
    d. ask questions to see if he understands or get a translator to explain
24. (Any 3 of the following) beliefs and practices regarding health and illness, language differences, eye contact, ways of dealing with terminal illness and/or severe disability, touch
25. subjective observations cannot be seen or felt, objective observations can be seen or measured
26. cross out neatly with a straight line, record "error," and initial
27. Health Insurance Portability and Accountability Act; establishes standards for maintaining confidentiality of health care records
28. many professionals with different levels of education, ideas, backgrounds, and interests working together for the benefit of the patient.
29. (Any 5 of the following) maintain a positive attitude, be friendly and cooperate with others, assist others when they need help, listen to others, respect opinions of others, be open-minded and willing to compromise, avoid criticizing others, learn good communication skills, support and encourage others, perform duties to the best of your ability
30. a. democratic: encourages participation of all individuals in a group, listens to opinions of others, bases decisions on what is best for the group as a whole
    b. laissez-faire: believes in noninterference, has minimal rules or regulations, allows individuals to function independently, avoids making decisions until forced to do so
    c. autocratic: dictator, maintains total rule, makes all decisions, has difficulty delegating or sharing duties, expects others to follow directions at all times.
31. body's reaction to any stimulus that requires a person to adjust to a changing environment
32. stop: break out of stress response; breathe: take slow, deep breaths to relieve physical tension; reflect: think about the problem at hand and the cause of stress; choose: determine how you want to deal with the stress
33. answers will be individualized; evaluate student's solutions to dealing with stress

34. short-term goals usually take days, weeks, or months to accomplish while long-term goals may take a period of years or a lifetime to accomplish; short-term goals are the smaller steps taken to reach long-term goals
35. (1) analyze and prioritize, (2) identify habits and preferences, (3) schedule tasks, (4) make a daily to-do list, (5) plan your work, (6) avoid distractions, (7) take credit for a job well done

CHAPTER 5 LEGAL AND ETHICAL RESPONSIBILITIES

1.
   a. CONTRACT
   b. TORTS
   c. SLANDER
   d. DEFAMATION
   e. LIBEL
   f. LEGAL DISABILITY
   g. LEGAL
   h. AGENT
   i. ETHICS
   j. FALSE IMPRISONMENT
   k. MALPRACTICE
   l. ASSAULT
   m. NEGLIGENCE
   n. PATIENTS RIGHTS

2. criminal law focuses on the wrongs against a person, property, or society; civil law focuses on the legal relationships between people and the protection of a person's rights
3. situations will be individualized; make sure the situation created brings out the following information:
   a. malpractice: failure of a professional to use the degree of skill and learning commonly expected in a profession
   b. negligence: failure to give care that is normally expected
   c. assault and battery: threat or attempt to injure or unlawful touching of another person without consent
   d. invasion of privacy: unnecessarily exposing an individual or revealing personal information about an individual without consent
   e. false imprisonment: restraining an individual or restricting an individual's freedom
   f. abuse: any care that results in physical harm, pain, or mental anguish
   g. defamation: false statements causing ridicule or damage
4. both refer to giving out incorrect information in error; slander is spoken, and libel is written
5. offer, acceptance, consideration
6. implied contracts cause obligations without verbally expressed terms; expressed contracts state in distinct and clear language either orally or in writing
7. (Any 3 of the following) minor, mentally incompetent persons, individuals under the influence of drugs that alter the mental state, semiconscious or unconscious persons
8. interpreter/translator must be provided
9. principal is responsible for the actions of an agent; principal may be required to compensate or pay people whom agent has injured
10. all information given to health care personnel by a patient; written consent of the patient
11. (Any 3 of the following) birth and death information, injuries caused by violence, drug abuse, communicable diseases, sexually transmitted diseases
12. health care provider; right to obtain a copy of any information in the record
13. cross out error with a single line so material is still readable, insert correct information, initial and date entry
14. (Any 3 of the following) limit personnel with access, use codes, require passwords, monitor and evaluate computer use
15. Standards for Privacy of Individually Identifiable Health Information as a result of HIPAA
16. identify the purpose or need for the information, extent of the information that may be released, limits on the release of the information, date of the authorization, signature of the person authorized to give consent
17. set of principles relating to what is morally right or wrong

18. a. report to immediate supervisor, b. report to immediate supervisor, c. refer question to dentist, d. report the signs to immediate supervisor or to individual responsible for reporting suspicions of abuse to proper authorities
19. patient's rights, considerate, respectful, information, informed, treatment, confidential, response, examine, explanation, participate, continuity
20. Omnibus Budget Reconciliation Act (OBRA) of 1987
21. a. Living will: allows an individual to state what measures should or should not be taken to prolong life when his or her condition is terminal
    b. Durable Power of Attorney (POA): permits an individual to appoint another person to make decisions regarding health care when the individual is unable to make decisions
22. requires all health care facilities receiving federal aid to inform every adult of his or her right to make decisions concerning medical care, including the right to refuse treatment and right-to-die options
23. (Any 2 of the following) check name band, state patient's name clearly, repeat name
24. a. state that you are not qualified or legally permitted to give injections
    b. check with immediate supervisor; do not take the temperature
    c. explain that you are not authorized to reveal the information and refer the wife to her husband's doctor or your supervisor
25. do not resuscitate order; means that CPR is not performed when the patient stops breathing

CHAPTER 6 MEDICAL TERMINOLOGY

CHAPTER 6:1 USING MEDICAL ABBREVIATIONS

A. Meanings of Abbreviations

1. discontinued, discharge
2. operating room
3. whenever necessary, as needed
4. before meals
5. immediately, at once
6. registered nurse
7. weight
8. chloride, chlorine
9. prescription, take, treatment
10. apical pulse
11. temperature
12. nothing by mouth
13. specimen
14. with
15. one-half
16. without
17. patient, pint
18. blood pressure
19. respiration, rectal
20. sodium
21. Centers for Disease Control and Prevention
22. diagnostic related group
23. last menstrual period
24. higher, elevate, up
25. female
26. venipuncture, venous pressure
27. automated external defibrillation
28. Health Insurance Portability and Accountability Act
29. long-term care
30. body mass index

B. Interpretation of Combined Abbreviations

1. temperature, pulse, and respiration four times a day
2. two drops twice a day
3. one cubic centimeter intramuscular
4. blood pressure every four hours
5. 2 ounces orange juice four times a day before meals and hour of sleep (bedtime)
6. weight and height every other day in morning (before noon)
7. bedrest with bathroom privileges only
8. 1000 milliliters normal saline intravenous
9. do electrocardiogram in coronary care unit
10. dissolve 2 teaspoons sodium chloride (salt) in 1 quart water
11. 1000 cubic centimeters soap solution enema at hour of sleep
12. schedule blood work in the morning (before noon) including complete blood count, blood urea nitrogen, and fasting blood sugar
13. dilute 1 tablet in one pint water
14. one capsule four times a day after meals and hour of sleep
15. blood pressure is measured in millimeters of mercury

16. nothing by mouth before an operation
17. do ear, eye, nose, and throat exam in outpatient department
18. obstetrics-gynecology
19. 500 milligrams every other day at 8 in the morning (before noon)
20. vital signs immediately (at once) and every two hours
21. to physical therapy by wheelchair for range-of-motion and activities of daily living twice a day
22. force fluids clear liquids to 240 milliliters every 2 hours
23. 2 drops each eye 4 times a day every 6 hours
24. diagnosis: chronic obstructive pulmonary disease, oxygen whenever necessary, intermittent positive pressure breathing twice a day every 12 hours
25. give the following directions: 2 capsules by mouth 3 times a day with food or milk
26. diagnosis: cerebral vascular accident, computerized tomography scan of the brain immediately (at once)
27. prescription: 20 milliliters potassium chloride intravenous
28. emergency medical technician is certified for advanced cardiac life support

CHAPTER 6:2 INTERPRETING WORD PARTS

A. Identifying Word Parts

1. cutting into the skull
2. difficult urination
3. surgical removal of the uterus
4. blood poisoning
5. inflammation around the heart
6. white cell
7. inflammation of the gallbladder
8. rapid heart
9. nerve pain
10. excess of blood cells
11. slow heart
12. surgical removal of the stomach
13. inflammation of membranes covering the brain and spinal cord
14. new disease
15. person who studies the skin
16. instrument for examining the rectum
17. malignant tumor, cancer
18. instrument for recording electrical activity of the brain
19. softening of a bone
20. paralysis of lower half of the body
21. pus in the urine
22. enlarged extremities
23. study of the elderly, old age
24. difficult or painful eating or swallowing
25. swelling or tumor of water

B. Analyzing Words

1. tumor of a gland
2. against poisons
3. study of the eye
4. surgical removal of the gallbladder
5. inflammation within the heart
6. inflammation of the stomach and intestine
7. low blood sugar
8. poison blood
9. less than normal urine (output)
10. inflammation of air tubes in the lungs
11. same kind or type
12. condition of hardening of the arteries
13. difficult or painful flow of menstruation
14. disease or abnormal condition of the vessels
15. sewing or suturing of the eyelid
16. inflammation of the urethra and bladder
17. condition of blackness in the lung
18. disease near a bone or joint
19. hernia of the fallopian tube and ovary
20. self-originating disease with a deficiency or decrease in the number of cells causing clot formation
21. seizure while sleeping
22. after birth
23. suture or sewing up of a rupture
24. condition of blueness of skin
25. surgical puncture to remove fluid from the thorax or chest

Note to Instructor: Use the abbreviation and word element lists to develop weekly tests. This provides the student with application of knowledge and provides a means of evaluation of this chapter.

CHAPTER 7 ANATOMY AND PHYSIOLOGY

CHAPTER 7:1 BASIC STRUCTURE OF THE HUMAN BODY

1. A. cell membrane: outer protective covering
   B. endoplasmic reticulum: transports materials in and out of nucleus, aids in synthesis and storage of protein
   C. nucleus: controls activities of cells
   D. nucleolus: reproduction of cell
   E. chromatin: forms chromosomes that contain genes
   F. cytoplasm: fluid containing water, food, and special materials; site for all chemical reactions in cell
   G. mitochondria: produce energy
   H. golgi apparatus: produces, stores, and packages secretions for discharge from the cell
   I. lysosomes: contain digestive enzymes to digest and destroy old cells, bacteria, and foreign materials
   J. pinocytic vesicle: allow protein or fat to enter cell
   k. vacuole: pouchlike structure filled with watery substance, stored food, or waste products
2. anatomy, physiology, pathophysiology
3. cell
4. (Any 4 of the following) take in food and oxygen, produce heat and energy, move and adapt to the environment, eliminate wastes, perform specific functions, reproduce
5. strings of DNA nucleotides
6. mitosis, see figure 7-2 in the textbook to evaluate the students' sketches
7. dehydration, edema
8. epithelial: covers surface of the body and lines body cavities
   connective: supporting fabric of organs and body parts
   nerve: controls and coordinates body activities by transmitting messages throughout the body
   muscle: produces power and movement
9. adipose
10. stores fat to provide energy, insulate the body, fill the area between tissue fibers, and provide padding for body
11. bone tissue has calcium salts, nerves, and blood vessels
12. skeletal: provides movement of the body
    cardiac: causes the heart to beat
    visceral or smooth: forms walls of the respiratory, digestive, urinary tract, and blood vessels
13. organ, heart, stomach, lungs
14. (Any 10 of the following) integumentary, skeletal, muscular, circulatory, lymphatic, nervous, special senses, respiratory, digestive, urinary, endocrine, reproductive

CHAPTER 7:2 BODY PLANES, DIRECTIONS, AND CAVITIES

1. (1) C (3) G (5) M (7) J (9) K (11) H (13) E
   (2) L (4) F (6) I (8) B (10) D (12) A
2. A. dorsal B. ventral C. cranial D. spinal E. thoracic F. abdominal G. pelvic H. orbital I. nasal J. buccal
3. cranial: brain
   spinal: spinal cord
   thoracic: esophagus, trachea, bronchi, lungs, heart, large blood vessels
   upper abdominal: stomach, small intestine, most of large intestine, appendix, liver, gallbladder, pancreas, spleen
   pelvic: urinary bladder, reproductive organs, last part of large intestines
   orbital: eyes
   nasal: nose structures
   buccal: teeth, tongue

4. right upper quadrant (RUQ), left upper quadrant (LUQ), right lower quadrant (RLQ), left lower quadrant (LLQ)
5. a. epigastric, b. right iliac/inguinal, c. left hypochondriac, d. umbilical, e. right lumbar, f. hypogastric or pelvic

CHAPTER 7:3 INTEGUMENTARY SYSTEM

1. A. epidermis
   B. dermis
   C. subcutaneous fascia or hypodermis
   D. dermal papilla
   E. sweat pore
   F. hair shaft
   G. strata corneum
   H. strata germinativum
   I. sebaceous (oil) gland
   J. hair follicle
   K. nerve fiber
   L. sudoriferous (sweat) gland
   M. artery
   N. vein
2. areas on dermis that fit into ridges on the strata germinativum; form an individual's unique fingerprints and footprints
3. sudoriferous; water, salts, body wastes
4. sebaceous; produce an oil that keeps skin and hair from becoming dry and brittle, help prevent infection
5. baldness or a permanent loss of hair on the scalp
6. protection, sensory perception, body temperature regulation, storage, absorption, excretion, production
7. dilate: get larger; excess heat escapes through the skin

   constrict: get smaller; heat is retained in the body
8. a. erythema: reddish color, caused by burns or congestion of blood in the vessels
   b. jaundice: yellow discoloration, presence of bile in the blood caused by liver or gallbladder disease or destruction of red blood cells
   c. cyanosis: bluish discoloration, caused by insufficient oxygen and seen with heart, lung, and circulatory diseases
9. a. vesicles, b. papules, c. crusts or scabs, d. pustules, e. macules, f. wheals, g. ulcer
10. a. impetigo: contagious skin infection characterized by yellow crusty sores
    b. verrucae: warts caused by a viral infection
    c. dermatitis: inflammation of the skin
    d. acne vulgaris: inflammation of sebaceous glands
    e. athlete's foot: contagious fungus infection that usually affects the feet
    f. psoriasis: chronic, noncontagious, inherited skin disease with red thick areas covered with white or silver scales
    g. ringworm: highly contagious fungus disease characterized by a flat or raised circular area with a clear center surrounded by an itchy, scaly, or crusty outer ring
    h. basal cell carcinoma: a cancer of the basal cells in the epidermis that grows slowly and usually does not spread
    i. melanoma: a cancer that develops in the melanocytes of the epidermis that spreads rapidly and is the most dangerous skin cancer

CHAPTER 7:4 SKELETAL SYSTEM

1. **Answers to crossword puzzle**

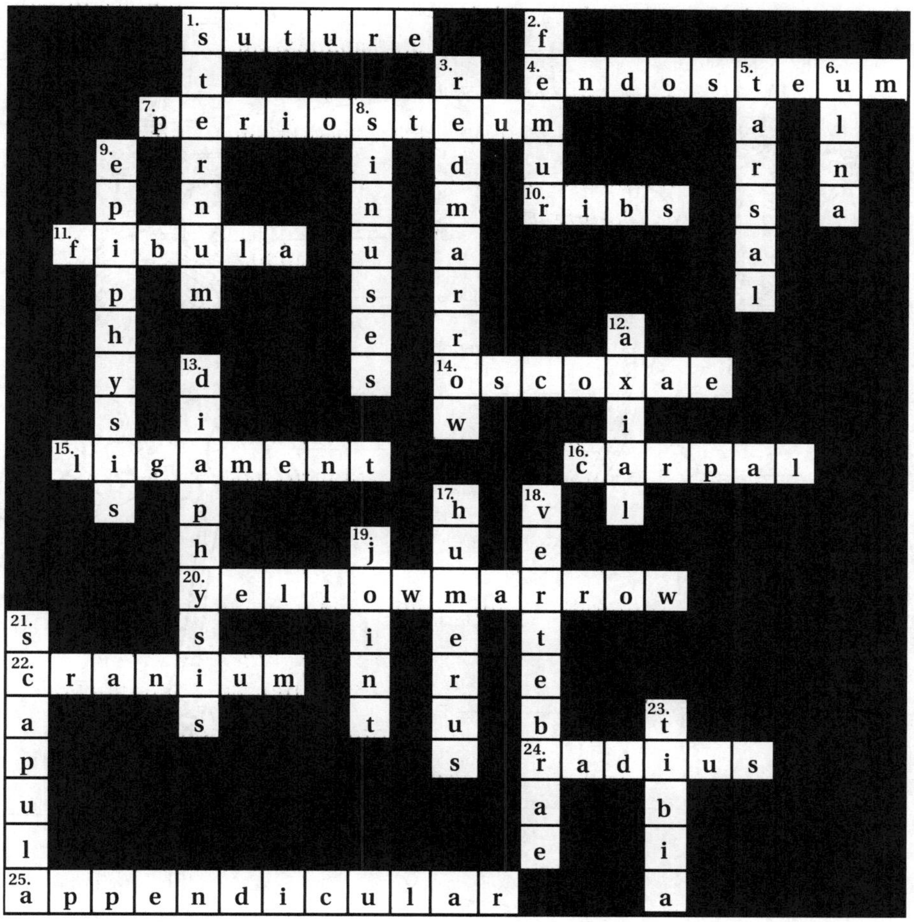

2. framework, protection, levers, produce blood cells, storage of calcium
3. frontal, two parietal, two temporal, occipital, ethmoid, sphenoid
4. seven cervical, twelve thoracic, five lumbar, sacrum, coccyx
5. true ribs attach to the sternum, false ribs attach with cartilage to the rib above, floating ribs have no attachment on the front of the body
6. xiphoid process
7. ilium, ischium, pubis
8. diarthrosis: freely movable, shoulder, hip, elbow, or knee

   amphiarthrosis: slightly movable, vetebrae and symphysis pubis

   synarthrosis: immovable, suture joints of cranium
9. connective tissue bands that hold bones together at joints
10. a. arthritis: group of diseases involving inflammation in the joints
    b. fractures: cracks or breaks in bone
    c. osteomyelitis: a bone inflammation usually caused by a pathogenic organism
    d. osteoporosis: disease in which bones become porous or soft and likely to fracture
    e. sprain: damage to ligaments in a joint
    f. bursitis: inflammation of small, fluid-filled sacs surrounding joints
    g. dislocation: bone is forcibly displaced from a joint
    h. scoliosis: side-to-side or lateral curvature of the spine

11. diagram of bones of a skeleton

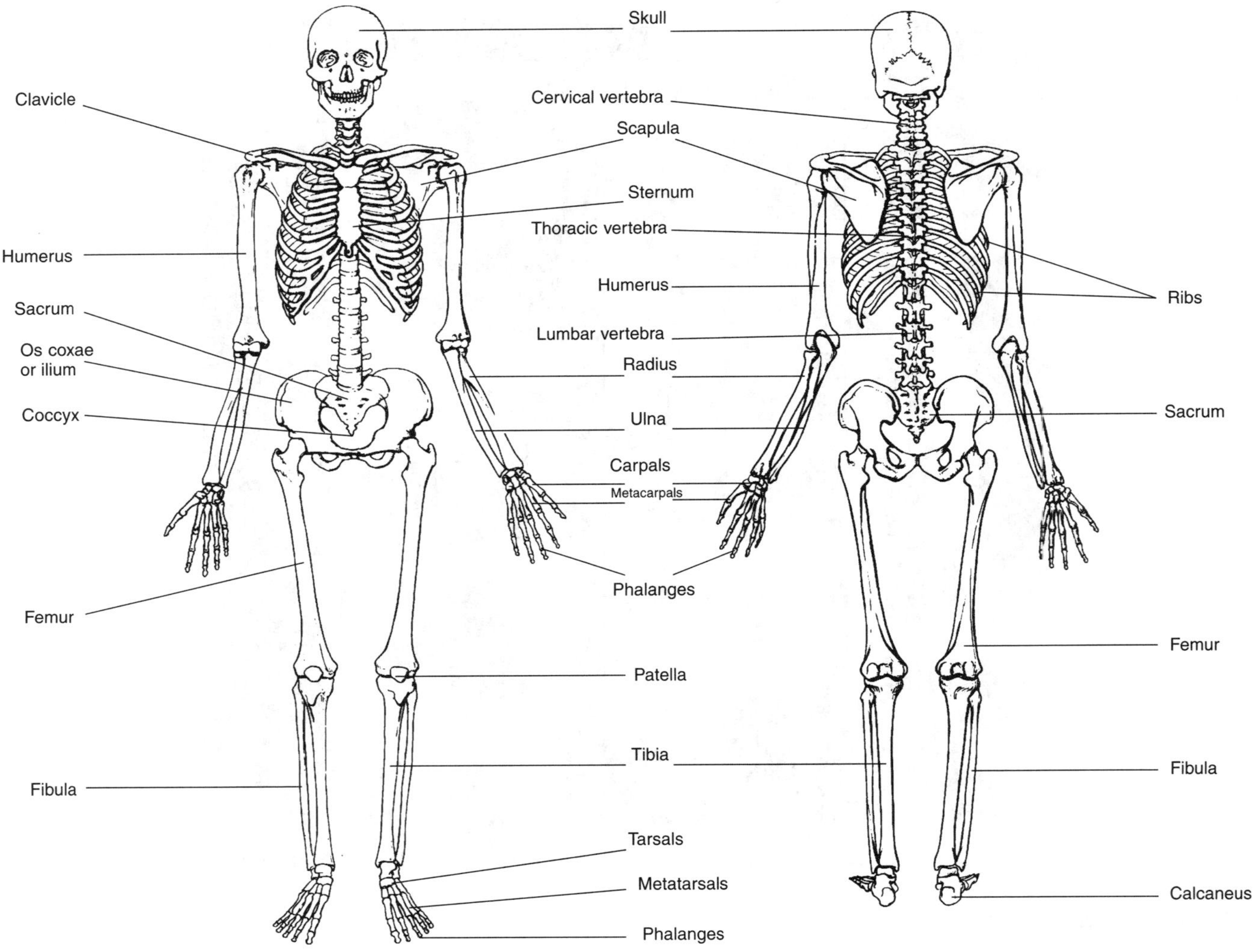

CHAPTER 7:5 MUSCULAR SYSTEM

1. a. excitability or irritability, b. extensibility, c. contractility, d. elasticity
2. cardiac: contract to circulate blood
   visceral or smooth: contract to cause movement in body systems
   skeletal: attach to bones and cause body movement
3. involuntary muscles: function without conscious thought or control
   voluntary muscles: person has control over their actions
4. voluntary movement, produce heat and energy, maintain posture, protect internal organs
5. tendon, fascia
6. a. flexion, b. circumduction, c. adduction, d. flexion, e. abduction, f. extension, g. extension, h. rotation, i. adduction, j. rotation
7. state of partial contraction
8. muscles waste away, lack of use
9. severe tightening of a flexor muscle resulting in bending of a joint; foot, fingers, wrist, and knees

10. a. biceps brachii; b. sartorius; c. trapezius; d. intercostals; e. tibialis anterior; f. gluteus maximus, quadriceps femoris, and deltoid; g. rectus abdominus; h. pectoralis major; i. sternocleidomastoid; j. quadriceps femoris

11. a. muscle spasms: sudden, painful, involuntary contractions of muscles
    b. muscular dystrophy: group of inherited diseases that leads to a chronic progressive muscle atrophy
    c. myasthenia gravis: chronic condition in which nerve impulses are not transmitted properly to the muscles
    d. strain: overstretching or injury to a muscle and/or tendon
    e. fibromyalgia: chronic widespread pain in specific muscle sites

CHAPTER 7:6 NERVOUS SYSTEM

1.

```
S E T P A R A S Y M P A T H E T I C M I U B E M S D
A V N E M R U R E N T H E C M R S E D T I C E I L W
T X Q R Z D E I U T E L C I R T N E V X L O V D E S
A I D I U L F L A N I P S O R B E R E C M M E B R F
G L O P Y D J O S E S H A R O L U O U I S E X R W T
N A N H N I A M A R K A R E C E R E B R U M C A E R
O E C E R E B E L L U M B R U M O S Y S T O M I T H
L I S R I S C R A Z E N A N D I N A M N O T S N U R
B E W A H Y I A M D O E I M G I D R O C L A N I P S
O T B L U T Y G U E S R S H A V U N R I C T K E O X
A C E N T R A L N E R V O U S S Y S T E M W O G N U
L L D E U N D E R B L E O O D L Y M P H E R Y N S P
L S B R A I N P I C I T E H T A P M Y S N A L I C O
U R D V N A T O P H Y S I O L E G E E R T S D N M I
D D I O V E R S I O C C F E D I P A Y T I O N E L J
E X A U T O N O M I C N E R V O U S S Y S T E M M H
M C A S Y S T E M N Y O U F I N D T H E W O R D S I
```

2. neuron, nucleus, dendrites, axon, myelin sheath, impulse, insulates, maintains
3. space between axon of a neuron and dendrites of other neurons
4. A. ventricles: hollow spaces that contain cerebrospinal fluid
   B. cerebrum: reasoning, thought, memory, speaking, sensation, sight, hearing, and voluntary body movement
   C. midbrain: conducts impulses between brain parts, eye reflex actions
   D. pons: conducts messages to other parts of brain; reflex actions such as respiration, chewing, tasting, and production of saliva
   E. cerebellum: coordination of muscles, balance, and posture; muscle tone
   F. medulla oblongata: regulates heartbeat, respiration, swallowing, coughing, and blood pressure
   G. spinal cord: reflex actions, carries sensory and motor messages
   H. meninges: cover and protect brain and spinal cord
5. dura mater, arachnoid membrane, pia mater; cover and protect the brain and spinal cord
6. shock absorber to protect the brain and spinal cord; carries nutrients and helps remove metabolic products and wastes
7. somatic, autonomic, cranial nerves, spinal nerves

8. sympathetic: increases heart rate, respiration, and blood pressure; decreases activity in digestive tract
   parasympathetic: decreases heart rate, respiration, and blood pressure; increases activity in digestive tract
9. balanced state in the body
10. a. paraplegia: paralysis of the lower extremities
    b. encephalitis: inflammation of the brain usually caused by a virus, bacteria, or chemical agent
    c. hydrocephalus: excessive accumulation of cerebrospinal fluid in the ventricles
    d. neuralgia: nerve pain
    e. cerebrovascular accident: stroke; damage to the brain resulting from a blood clot or hemorrhage
    f. epilepsy: condition involving abnormal electrical impulses in the brain resulting from seizures or convulsions
    g. cerebral palsy: disturbance in voluntary muscle action caused by brain damage
    h. Parkinson's disease: chronic progressive condition involving degeneration of brain cells
    i. amyotrophic lateral sclerosis: chronic degenerative neuromuscular disease

CHAPTER 7:7 SPECIAL SENSES

1. sensations, brain, interprets, responds
2. A. sclera: outermost tough connective tissue layer of the eye
   B. choroid: middle layer of the eye; nourishes the eye
   C. retina: innermost nerve-sensitive layer of the eye
   D. conjunctiva: mucous membrane that covers and protects the eye
   E. cornea: allows light rays to enter the eye
   F. aqueous humor: maintains forward curvature of the eyeball and bends or refracts light rays
   G. iris: muscle that controls the size of the pupil
   H. pupil: hole in the choroid coat that allows light rays to enter
   I. lens: refracts light rays
   J. vitreous humor: maintains shape of the eyeball and refracts light rays
3. bony socket of skull, eyelids and eyelashes, lacrimal glands, conjunctiva
4. cornea, aqueous humor, pupil, lens, vitreous humor; vision is distorted or blurred
5. a. astigmatism, b. glaucoma, c. myopia, d. strabismus, e. cataract, f. conjunctivitis, g. presbyopia, h. macular degeneration
6. wax produced in the outer ear; protects the ear
7. tympanic membrane; vibrates when sound waves hit it and transmits waves to the middle ear
8. malleus, incus, stapes
9. tube between the middle ear and throat; equalizes air pressure on both sides of the tympanic membrane
10. a. vestibule: acts as an entrance to two other parts of the inner ear
    b. cochlea: contains the organ of Corti
    c. organ of Corti: transmits sound impulses to the auditory nerve
    d. semicircular canals: send impulses that are interpreted as the sense of balance and equilibrium
11. otitis media, otosclerosis, conduction, sensory
12. sweet and salty at tip, sour at sides, and bitter at back of tongue
13. olfactory receptors
14. (Any 4 of the following) pressure, heat, cold, touch, pain

CHAPTER 7:8 CIRCULATORY SYSTEM

1. Answers to crossword puzzle

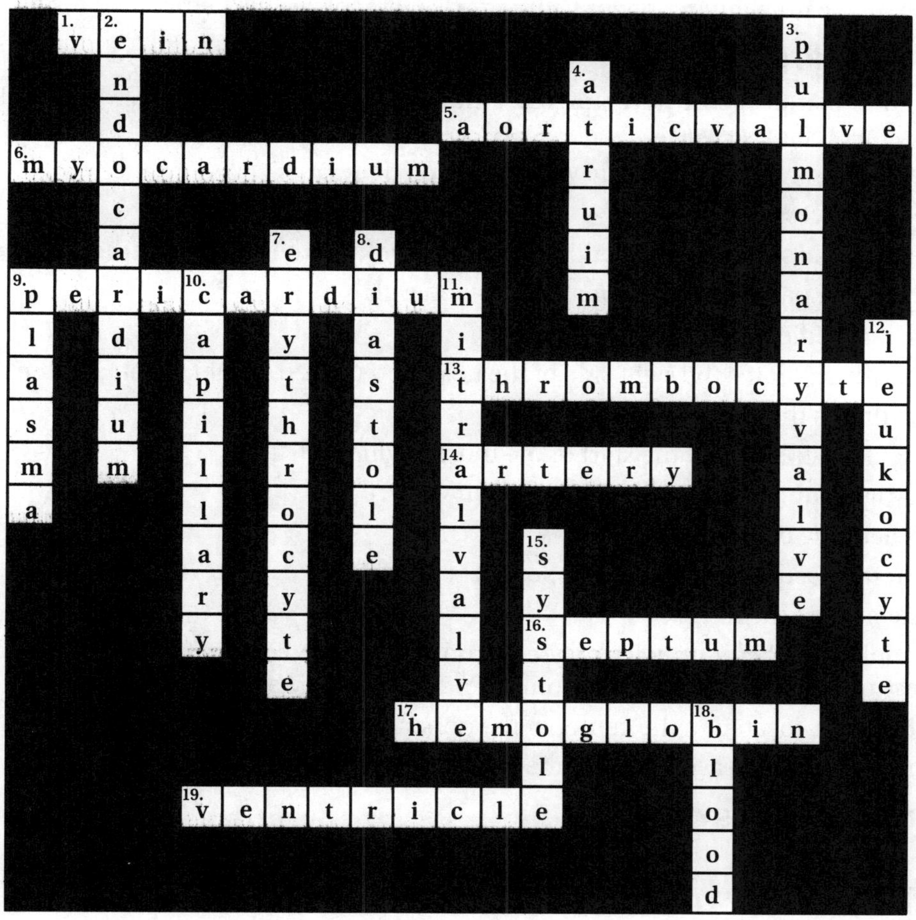

2. A. pericardium
   B. myocardium
   C. endocardium
   D. septum
   E. superior vena cava
   F. inferior vena cava
   G. right atrium
   H. tricuspid valve
   I. right ventricle
   J. pulmonary semilunar valve
   K. pulmonary artery
   L. pulmonary veins
   M. left atrium
   N. bicuspid or mitral valve
   O. left ventricle
   P. aortic semilunar valve
   Q. aorta
3. diastole: atria contract and push blood into the ventricles
4. systole: right ventricle pushes blood into the pulmonary artery so blood goes to the lungs, left ventricle pushes blood into the aorta so blood goes to all parts of the body
5. sinoatrial (SA) node, pathways in atria, atrioventricular (AV) node, bundle of His, right and left bundle branches, Purkinje fibers
6. abnormal heart rhythm; cardiac monitors and electrocardiogram
7. a. arteries, b. veins, c. capillaries, d. aorta, e. superior and inferior vena cava, f. capillaries, g. arterioles, h. venules, i. veins, j. arteries
8. oxygen, carbon dioxide, nutrients, metabolic waste products, heat, hormones
9. (Any 6 of the following) blood proteins, nutrients, mineral salts, vitamins, gases, metabolic waste products, hormones, enzymes
10. erythrocytes: 4.5 to 5.5 million, carry oxygen and carbon dioxide
    leukocytes: 5,000 to 9,000, fight infection
    thrombocytes: 250,000 to 400,000, aid in the clotting process
11. hemoglobin and the amount of oxygen present
12. complex protein found on red blood cells; carries oxygen and carbon dioxide

13. a. neutrophils and/or monocytes, b. lymphocytes, c. eosinophils, d. basophils
14. a. aneurysm; b. anemias; c. varicose veins; d. atherosclerosis; e. hemophilia; f. hypertension; g. thrombophlebitis; h. myocardial infarction, or heart attack; i. embolus; j. leukemia

CHAPTER 7:9 LYMPHATIC SYSTEM

1. thin watery fluid; composed of water, digested nutrients, salts, hormones, oxygen, carbon dioxide, lymphocytes, and metabolic wastes
2. lymphatic capillaries, lymph, lymphatic vessels, lymph nodes
3. valves in the lymph vessels
4. specialized lymphatic capillaries; pick up digested fats or lipids and transport them to the bloodstream
5. carbon, cancer cells, pathogens or germs, dead blood cells
6. lymphocytes, antibodies
7. right lymphatic duct: drains the right side of the head and neck, the right chest, and the right arm
   thoracic duct: drains the rest of the body
8. enlarged pouchlike structure at the start of the thoracic duct
9. bloodstream, right subclavian vein, left subclavian vein
10. palatine: on each side of the soft palate
    pharyngeal: in the nasopharynx on the upper part of the throat
    lingual: on the back of the tongue
11. (Any 4 of the following) produces leukocytes, produces antibodies, destroys old erythrocytes, stores erythrocytes, destroys thrombocytes, filters some metabolites and wastes from tissues
12. mass of lymph tissue located in the center of the upper chest; atrophies or wastes away after puberty
13. a. adenitis, b. Hodgkin's disease, c. splenomegaly, d. tonsillitis, e. lymphangitis

CHAPTER 7:10 RESPIRATORY SYSTEM

1. A. nostrils
   B. nasal cavity
   C. sinuses
   D. pharynx
   E. esophagus
   F. epiglottis
   G. larynx
   H. trachea
   I. left lung
   J. right lung
   K. right and left bronchi
   L. bronchiole
   M. alveolus
2. warmed, filtered, moistened
3. tiny hairlike structures that filter inhaled air to trap dust and other particles in the mucus; they then help move the mucus to the esophagus so it can be swallowed
4. nasopharynx, oropharynx, laryngopharynx
5. air leaves the lungs, and the vocal cords in the larynx vibrate to produce sound; tongue and lips act on sound to produce speech
6. epiglottis
7. blood capillaries, oxygen, carbon dioxide, surfactant
8. the heart lies more to the left side of the chest
9. a. inspiration: diaphragm and intercostal muscles contract and enlarge the thoracic cavity; air rushes in through the air tubes to the alveoli
   b. expiration: diaphragm and intercostal muscles relax, and air is forced out of the lungs and air passages
10. external respiration is the exchange of oxygen and carbon dioxide between the lungs and bloodstream; internal respiration is the exchange of oxygen and carbon dioxide between the bloodstream and tissue cells

11. tissue cells use oxygen and nutrients to produce energy, water, and carbon dioxide
12. decreased amount of oxygen or increased amounts of carbon dioxide in the blood
13. BRONCHITIS
    INFLUENZA
    SINUSITIS
    EMPHYSEMA
    EPISTAXIS
    TUBERCOULOSIS
    ASTHMA
    RHINITIS
    COPD
    PLEURISY
    LARYNGITIS
14. continuous positive airway pressure; used to deliver pressure to keep the airway open on individuals who have sleep apnea
15. possible diseases caused by smoking include bronchitis, COPD, emphysema, and lung cancer; evaluate student's individual answers on ways to quit smoking

UNIT 7:11 DIGESTIVE SYSTEM

1. A. mouth or oral cavity
   B. salivary glands
   C. pharynx
   D. esophagus
   E. liver
   F. gallbladder
   G. stomach
   H. pancreas
   I. duodenum
   J. jejunum
   K. ileum
   L. cecum
   M. vermiform appendix
   N. ascending colon
   O. transverse colon
   P. descending colon
   Q. sigmoid colon
   R. rectum
2. tastes food, aids with chewing and swallowing of food
3. chewing and grinding of food by the teeth
4. parotid, sublingual, submandibular, lubricates, moistens, salivary amylase, carbohydrates, starches, bolus
5. peristalsis
6. (Any 4 of the following) food converted to chyme; hydrochloric acid kills bacteria, helps in absorption of iron, helps activate the enzyme pepsin; rennin digests milk in infants; lipase starts the chemical breakdown of fats; pepsin starts protein digestion
7. a. maltase: breaks down sugars into simpler forms
   b. sucrase: breaks down sugars into simpler forms
   c. peptidases: complete the digestion of proteins
   d. bile: emulsifies or physically breaks down fats
   e. pancreatic amylase or amylopsin: chemically breaks down sugars
   f. trypsin: chemically breaks down proteins
   g. lipase or steapsin: chemically breaks down fats
8. villi, blood capillaries, lacteals, digested nutrients, fats
9. (Any 3 of the following) absorption of water and remaining nutrients, storage of indigestible materials, transportation of waste products, synthesis and absorption of some B-complex vitamins and vitamin K
10. ascending colon, transverse colon, descending colon, sigmoid colon
11. (Any 5 of the following) secretes bile, stores sugar or glycogen, stores iron, stores vitamins, produces heparin, produces fibrinogen and prothrombin, produces cholesterol, detoxifies substances
12. stores and concentrates bile
13. pancreas; produces pancreatic juice with enzymes to digest food and produces insulin to regulate metabolism of carbohydrates
14. a. hepatitis, b. diarrhea, c. cholelithiasis, d. cirrhosis, e. hemorrhoids, f. ulcerative colitis, g. gastroenteritis, h. hiatal hernia

15. type A hepatitis is transmitted in food or water contaminated by the feces of an infected person; type B hepatitis is transmitted by body fluids including blood, serum, saliva, urine, semen, vaginal secretions, and breast milk; type C hepatitis also is transmitted through contact with blood or body fluids; health care workers can contact the virus through contaminated body fluids and must take precautions to prevent the spread of these diseases

CHAPTER 7:12 URINARY SYSTEM

1. A. renal artery
   B. renal vein
   C. kidney
   D. renal cortex
   E. renal medulla
   F. renal pelvis or basin
   G. ureter
   H. urinary bladder
   I. urethra
   J. urinary meatus
2. a state of equilibrium, or constant state of natural balance in the internal environment of the body
3. nephrons, renal, glomerulus, water, mineral salts, glucose (sugar), metabolic products, Bowman's capsule, convoluted tubule, reabsorbed, capillaries, glucose, mineral salts, water, wastes, urine
4. peristalsis; moves urine from the kidney to the bladder
5. series of folds on the walls of the bladder; allow bladder to expand to fill with urine
6. females: urethra shorter and carries only urine

   males: longer and carries both urine and semen
7. urea, uric acid, creatinine, mineral salts, various pigments
8. a. polyuria: excessive urination
   b. oliguria: below normal amounts of urination
   c. anuria: absence of urination
   d. hematuria: blood in the urine
   e. pyuria: pus in the urine
   f. nocturia: urination at night
   g. dysuria: painful urination
   h. retention: inability to empty the bladder
   i. incontinence: involuntary urination
   j. proteinuria: protein in the urine
   k. albuminuria: albumin (a blood protein) in the urine
9. pyelonephritis, cystitis, renal calculi, uremia
10. removal of waste products from the blood by a hemodialysis machine
11. (Any 2 of the following) chromic glomerulonephritis, chronic renal failure, uremia

CHAPTER 7:13 ENDOCRINE SYSTEM

1. substances produced and secreted by endocrine glands; chemical messengers, transported by the blood stream
2. (Any 5 of the following) stimulate exocrine glands, stimulate endocrine glands, regulate growth and development, regulate metabolism, maintain fluid and chemical balance, control various sex processes
3. a. adrenal, b. ovaries, c. pituitary, d. thyroid, e. testes, f. parathyroids, g. pancreas
4. a. insulin, b. lactogenic or prolactin, c. somatotrophin, d. parathormone, e. testosterone, f. thyroxine, g. thyrotrophin, h. epinephrine or adrenalin, i. vasopressin, j. mineralocorticoids, k. estrogens, l. progesterone
5. (1) B (2) A (3) D (4) E (5) A (6) D (7) C (8) E (9) D (10) E
6. mass of tissue in the upper part of the chest; activates cells in the immune system in early life
7. placenta; expelled as the afterbirth
8. small structure located in the brain; produces melatonin, adrenoglomerulotropin, and serotonin
9. testes, ovaries
10. (Any 6 of the following) hyperglycemia, polyuria, polydipsia, polyphagia, glycosuria, weight loss, fatigue, slow healing of skin infections, vision changes

CHAPTER 7:14 REPRODUCTIVE SYSTEM

1. A. scrotum: sac suspended outside the body, contains the testes
   B. testes: produce sperm and the male hormone testosterone

   C. epididymis: stores sperm while they mature and become motile; also produces a fluid that becomes part of the semen
   D. ductus or vas deferens: passageway and temporary storage area for sperm
   E. seminal vesicle: produces thick yellow fluid that provides nourishment for the sperm
   F. ejaculatory duct: carries sperm and semen
   G. prostate gland: produces an alkaline secretion; contracts during ejaculation to empty the semen into the urethra
   H. urethra: carries urine from the bladder and semen from the reproductive tubes
   I. glans penis: enlarged structure at the distal end of the penis covered with the prepuce
   J. penis: male organ of copulation

2. the temperature is lower, which is ideal for the production of sperm
3. epididymis, seminal vesicles, prostate gland, Cowper's gland
4. vas deferens
5. circumcision
6. early detection of cancer in the testes; monthly
7. A. ovary: produce the ovum and female hormones
   B. fimbriae: help move the ovum into the fallopian tube
   C. infundibulum (uterine) or fallopian tube: passageway for the ovum from the ovary to the uterus; also the area for fertilization
   D. fundus of uterus: top section where the fallopian tubes attach
   E. uterine cavity or body of uterus: organ of menstruation, allows for the development of an infant, and aids in expulsion of the fetus during birth
   F. cervix of uterus: connects the uterus with the vagina
   G. vagina: passageway for menstrual flow, receives sperm, female organ of copulation, acts as the birth canal during delivery of an infant
8. union of the ovum with sperm to create a new life; takes place in the fallopian tube
9. peristalsis and cilia
10. endometrium; deteriorates and causes bleeding known as menstruation
11. vulva, labia majora, enclose, protect, labia minora, clitoris
12. detect breast tumors early; every month, at the end of menstruation, or on a scheduled day of the month after menopause
13. (Any 4 of the following) follow standard precautions, avoid high-risk sexual activities, use protective barrier during intercourse, avoid use of drugs and sharing of intravenous needles, avoid pregnancy if infected
14. Answers to crossword puzzle

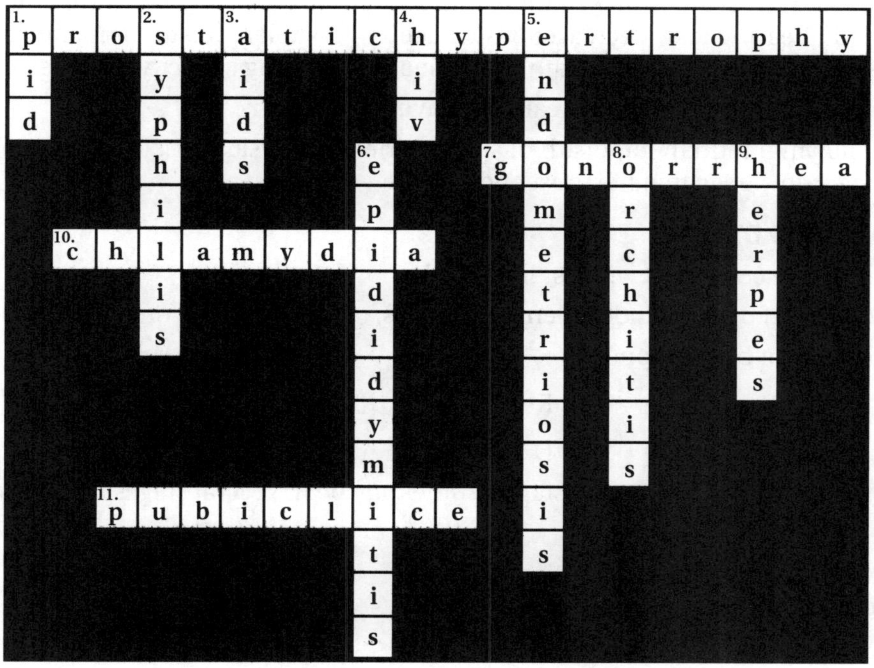

CHAPTER 8 HUMAN GROWTH AND DEVELOPMENT

CHAPTER 8:1 LIFE STAGES

1. growth refers to measurable physical changes that occur throughout an individual's life; development is more difficult to measure because it refers to changes in intellectual, mental, emotional, social, and functional skills
2. a. physical: body growth, height and weight changes, muscle and nerve development, changes in body organs
   b. mental or cognitive: intellectual development of mind; solve problems, make judgments, deal with situations
   c. emotional: feelings; dealing with love, hate, joy, fear, excitement
   d. social: interactions and relationships with others
3. a. Moro, or startle; b. rooting; c. sucking; d. grasp
4. a. 2–4 months, b. 6–8 months, c. 12 months, d. 6 months, e. 4–6 months, f. 6 months, g. 12 months
5. a. 2–4 years, b. 4 years, c. 6 years, d. 1–2 years, e. 6 years, f. 6 years
6. children like routines; become stubborn, angry, and frustrated when changes occur
7. loyalty, honesty, values, morals
8. development of sexual organs and secondary sexual characteristics
9. (Any 3 of the following) feel uncertain and inadequate and insecure; respond to peer group influences; changes in attitude and behavior; conflict with values previously established; worry about appearance, ability, and relationships with others
10. a. anorexia nervosa, b. bulimia, c. bulimarexia
11. (Any 4 of the following) anxiety or stress relief, peer pressure, escape from emotional or psychological problems, experimentation with feelings that chemicals produce, instant gratification, hereditary traits, cultural influences
12. no; individual is calling for help and needs support and understanding; otherwise, individual may commit suicide
13. (Any 5 of the following) education, dealing with independence, making career choices, determining life styles, selecting marital partner, starting a family, establishing values
14. satisfaction: (any 3 of the following) job stability, financial success, end of child rearing, good health; stress: (any 3 of the following) loss of job, fear of aging, loss of youth and vitality, illness, marital problems, problems with children/aging parents
15. (Any 8 of the following) skin becomes dry, wrinkled, and thin; brown or yellow spots appear; hair becomes thin and loses luster; bones become more brittle and porous; cartilage in vertebrae thins; muscles lose tone and strength; hearing loss; decreased visual acuity; less tolerance to temperature; memory loss; circulation decreases; kidney and bladder are less efficient; breathing capacity decreases
16. no; some much later because of better health and living conditions
17. (Any 4 of the following) retirement, death of spouse/friends, physical disabilities, financial problems, loss of independence, knowledge that life must end

CHAPTER 8:2 DEATH AND DYING

1. disease that cannot be cured that will result in death
2. (Any 3 of the following) pain, abandonment, loneliness, unknown, loved ones, unfinished work or dreams
3. should, some hope, not be left alone
4. (1) D (3) B (5) E (7) A–E (9) A and E (11) E
   (2) C (4) A (6) D (8) C (10) D (12) B
5. no; some may not progress through all stages, some may be in several stages at the same time, some may overlap
6. personal feelings, terms
7. allow patient to die with dignity and comfort

8. (Any 3 of the following) psychological, spiritual, social, and financial counseling; personal care; free or less expensive pain medication; pain control; volunteer support; contact with family after the death of the patient
9. advance directives
10. answers will be individualized; make sure students explain why they do or do not believe in the "right to die"
11. encourages people to make their end-of-life wishes known
12. answers will be individualized; make sure students name two rights from the Dying Person's Bill of Rights and explain why those rights are most important

CHAPTER 8:3 HUMAN NEEDS

1. lower needs should be met before an individual can strive for higher needs
2. food, water, oxygen, elimination of waste materials, sleep, protection from temperature extremes
3. (Any 3 of the following) new environment, change in routine, marital problems, loss of a job, injury or disease
4. fear for personal safety is more important than money and prestige
5. accept and adapt, unknown situations
6. (Any 3 of the following) friends are made, social contacts are established, acceptance by others is received, able to give and receive affection and love
7. people's feelings concerning their masculine/feminine nature, abilities to give and receive love and affection, roles in reproduction of the species
8. married couples may share the same room
9. when others show respect, approval, and appreciation
10. people have obtained their full potential or they are what they want to be
11. motivated, satisfaction, tension
12. hard work: work hard to get good grades to obtain a scholarship

    realistic goals: work as a respiratory therapy assistant to earn money for the education; consider a state college with a less expensive program

    evaluate situation: evaluate costs at other schools, obtain a job to help cover expenses, learn to budget and save money

    cooperate with others: live at home, share travel expenses with others, share books, find someone to sponsor education
13. unhealthy if used all of the time, healthy if aware of use and used to cope with certain situations
14. Situations will be individualized. Basic situations should show:
    a. rationalization: reasonable excuse or acceptable explanation for behavior
    b. projection: placing blame on someone else or circumstances
    c. displacement: transferring feelings about one person to someone else
    d. compensation: substitution of one goal for another goal
    e. daydreaming: escape to daydreaming, either good or bad
    f. repression: transfer of unacceptable or painful ideas, feelings, and thoughts into unconscious mind
    g. suppression: refusing to deal with unacceptable feelings or thoughts
    h. denial: disbelief of an event that is too frightening to cope with
    i. withdrawal: cease to communicate or remove self physically from a situation
15. Answers will be individualized. Basic answers should include:
    a. anger caused by lack of food/drink, fear of test or illness
    b. let patient express anger, explain purpose of test and why it takes so long, make every attempt to make patient as comfortable as possible, provide encouragement and support

CHAPTER 9 CULTURAL DIVERSITY

1. values, beliefs, attitudes, languages, symbols, rituals, behaviors, and customs unique to a particular group of people and passed from one generation to the next
2. learned, shared, social in nature and dynamic and constantly changing
3. ethnicity, race, cultural diversity
4. answers will be individualized, but students should state one of the following views:

   yes; cultural differences are recognized and respected

   no; cultural groups are forced to accept beliefs and behaviors of dominant society
5. a. stereotype, b. bias, c. prejudice, d. stereotype, e. prejudice, f. bias
6. (Any 6 of the following) know and be consciously aware of your own personal and professional values and beliefs; obtain as much information as possible about different ethnic/cultural groups; be sensitive to behaviors and practices different from your own; remember that you are not being pressured to adopt other beliefs but that you must respect them; develop friendships with a wide variety of people from different ethnic/cultural groups; ask and encourage questions; evaluate all information before you form an opinion; be open about differences; avoid ethnic or sexual jokes; remember that mistakes happen
7. care that provides for the well-being of the whole person and meets physical, social, emotional, and mental needs
8. (Any 5 of the following) family organization, language, personal space, touching, eye contact, gestures, health care beliefs, spirituality, religion
9. a. patriarchal, b. nuclear, c. extended, d. matriarchal
10. a. Asian
    b. Hispanic
    c. South African, Asian, and Native American
    d. Asian and Hispanic
    e. South African, Asian, Hispanic, Middle Eastern, and Native American
    f. South African, European, and Middle Eastern
    g. Asian
    h. South African, Middle Eastern, and Native American
    i. Middle Eastern
    j. Native American
    k. South African and European
11. no; spirituality is an individualized and personal set of beliefs and practices, religion is an organized system of belief
12. some religions require last rites, and religious representatives must be notified when death is imminent
13. Christian Scientists and Jehovah's Witnesses
14. atheist, agnostic
15. (Any 8 of the following) listen to patients as they express beliefs; learn to appreciate differences in people; learn about cultural and ethnic groups; recognize and avoid bias, prejudice, and stereotyping; ask questions to determine beliefs; evaluate all information before forming an opinion; allow patients to practice and express their beliefs; remember that you are not expected to adopt other's beliefs, just accept and respect them; recognize and promote patients' interactions with their families; be sensitive to patient's response to eye contact, touch, and invasion of personal space; respect spirituality, religious beliefs, symbols, and rituals
16. answers will be individualize but should contain information such as:
    a. try to find a translator (relative or other staff member) or check to see if you have written instructions in patient's language
    b. talk with physician to see if husband can be in the room
    c. talk with patient to find out significance of necklace; check with immediate supervisor or surgeon to see if necklace can be left on patient or taped in place to avoid being lost
    d. proceed at a slower pace; talk with patient and explain procedure while encouraging patient to relax; step back periodically to give patient "breathing room"; try to limit direct contact with patient as much as possible
    e. talk with patient and ask about daughter and family; find out if this is a usual routine; check with immediate supervisor to obtain permission for daughter to assist with bath

CHAPTER 10 GERIATRIC CARE

CHAPTER 10:1 MYTHS ON AGING

1. fact
2. myth: largest percentage remain mentally competent until they die
3. fact
4. fact
5. myth: financial situation of elderly varies just as financial situation of other age groups varies; less than 10 percent live at the poverty level
6. myth: most elderly individuals live with someone and/or associate frequently with friends and family members
7. myth: many people are employed and productive into their 70s and 80s
8. myth: "old" is not determined by the number of years lived as much as by how an individual thinks, feels, and behaves
9. fact
10. myth: many retired people enjoy full and active lives

CHAPTER 10:2 PHYSICAL CHANGES OF AGING

1. gradual, long period, rate, degree, lifestyle, nutrition, economic, social, normal, adapt, cope
2. (Any 3 of the following for each body system)
   a. integumentary: skin less elastic and dry; itching; senile lentigines; lines and wrinkles develop; nails become thick, tough, and brittle; sensitivity to temperature
   b. musculoskeletal: muscles lose tone, volume, and strength; bones become brittle and more likely to fracture; joints become stiff, less flexible, and painful; rib cage becomes rigid; vertebrae compress; slower movement; falls occur easily
   c. circulatory: cardiac output decreases, blood vessels narrow and become less elastic, blood flow to brain and other organs may decrease, blood pressure may increase
   d. respiratory: respiratory muscles weaker, rib cage more rigid, alveoli thinner and less elastic and exchange of gases decreases, bronchioles lose elasticity, changes in larynx cause higher-pitched and weaker voice
   e. nervous: progressive loss of brain cells; senses of taste, smell, vision, and hearing diminish; nerve endings less sensitive; decreased ability to respond to pain and stimuli; memory loss
   f. digestive: fewer digestive juices and enzymes produced, peristalsis decreases, teeth are lost, liver function reduced, dysphagia may develop, decreased taste sensation
   g. urinary: kidneys decrease in size and become less efficient, loss of ability to concentrate urine, ability of bladder to hold urine decreases, retention of urine occurs, nocturia and incontinence may occur
   h. endocrine: increased production of parathormone and thyroid-stimulating hormone, decreased production of other hormones, less efficient immune system, decreased basal metabolic rate, intolerance to glucose
   i. reproductive: decreased vaginal secretions, uterus sags downward, breasts sag, decreased production of sperm, sexual stimulation slower, testes get smaller and less firm, decreased seminal fluid
3. a. osteoporosis, b. arthritis, c. thrombus, d. emphysema, e. cataracts, f. glaucoma, g. dysphagia, h. incontinence, i. senile lentigines
4. a. use bath oils or moisturizing lotions, decrease daily baths
   b. set room temperature higher; use socks, sweaters, lap blankets, and layers of clothing
   c. avoid fluids in evening, rest during the day
   d. replace buttons with self-stick bands or strips
   e. install grab bars in bathroom and put stool in tub
   f. use two or three pillows, position in semi-Fowlers, avoid polluted air
   g. serve foods with variety of textures and tastes, carefully use seasonings
   h. encourage shorter exercise periods, alternate rest and exercise
   i. talk slowly and clearly, face individual, avoid yelling, eliminate background noise
   j. make regular trips to bathroom, wear easy-to-remove clothing, use absorbent pads

CHAPTER 10:3 PSYCHOSOCIAL CHANGES OF AGING

1. frustration, mental distress
2. (Any 2 of the following) part-time or consultant job, volunteer work, community or club activities
3. lose social contacts, feel useless, experience financial difficulties
4. (Any 2 of the following) children marry and move away, spouse dies, friends and relatives die
5. (Any 2 of the following) make new friends, establish new social contacts, participate in church and community groups
6. feel a loss of independence and become frightened by lack of control over environment
7. (Any 2 of the following) called "resident"; bring favorite pieces of furniture, pictures, television, and personal items; allow choice in arrangement of items
8. physical disabilities, illness, decreased mental ability
9. encourage patient to do as much as possible and make choices but provide for patient's safety
10. disease is any condition that interferes with normal function of body, and disability is a physical or mental defect or handicap that interferes with normal function
11. death, chronic illness, loss of function, pain
12. (Any 2 of the following) listen as the person expresses fears, be patient and understanding, provide supportive care

CHAPTER 10:4 CONFUSION AND DISORIENTATION IN THE ELDERLY

1. (Any 6 of the following) talking incoherently, not knowing name or not recognizing others, wandering aimlessly, displaying hostile and combative behavior, hallucinating, regressing in behavior, decreasing attention to personal hygiene, unable to respond to commands or follow instructions
2. (Any 6 of the following) stress, depression, alcohol, chemicals, kidney disease, respiratory disease, liver disease, medications, poor nutrition, lack of fluid intake
3. a. cerebrovascular accident or stroke, b. arteriosclerosis, c. atherosclerosis
4. chronic has permanent, irreversible damage to brain cells; delirium (acute dementia) has a treatable cause
5. a. middle, b. terminal, c. terminal, d. early, e. middle, f. terminal, g. early, h. middle, i. middle
6. safe, secure, routine, simple, noises, crowded, commotion, reality orientation
7. (answers will vary; some examples are given)
   a hang large clock in room
   b. keep room well lit and curtains open, wear regular clothes in daytime, provide activities to keep patient active during day
   c. call by correct name
   d. correctly identify yourself frequently
   e. put picture of patient on his/her door
   f. make sure hearing aid is in good working order, talk slowly and clearly
8. a. T b. T c. T d. F e. F f. F g. F h. F i. T j. T

CHAPTER 10:5 MEETING THE NEEDS OF THE ELDERLY

1. physical, psychological, physical, psychosocial
2. language, food habits, dress, work, leisure activities, health care
3. religion, bias, religious beliefs
4. (Any 3 of the following) allow patient to express feelings and thoughts, treat religious articles properly, allow person to practice his or her religion, honor requests for special foods, provide privacy during clergy visits
5. physical, verbal, psychological, sexual
6. verbal, physical, and psychological abuse; report it to your supervisor immediately
7. verbal, physical, and psychological abuse; report your observations to the physician immediately

8. want to protect abuser who may be family member or caretaker or believe they deserve abuse
9. ensure the elderly individual of "kind and considerate care" and provide for meeting individual needs
10. Ombudsman, investigate, resolve, improvements, monitor, enforce, problems, education

CHAPTER 11 NUTRITION AND DIETS

A. Matching

1. M	3. J	5. E	7. F	9. B
2. H	4. D	6. N	8. A	10. P

B. Completion and Short Answer

1. (Any 4 of the following) healthy appearance, well-developed body, good attitude, proper sleep and bowel habits, high energy level, enthusiasm, freedom from anxiety
2. osteoporosis
3. cellulose
4. (Any 4 of the following) provide the most concentrated form of energy, provide insulation, cushion organs and bones, aid in absorption of fat-soluble vitamins, provide flavor
5. saturated are solid at room temperature, and polyunsaturated are soft or oily; a. (any 4 of the following) meats, eggs, whole milk, cream, butter, cheese; b. (any 3 of the following) vegetable oils, margarines, products made from vegetable oils, fish, peanuts
6. build and repair tissue, regulate body functions, produce energy and heat; complete proteins contain nine essential amino acids, whereas incomplete proteins contain some of the nine essential amino acids and any of the remaining thirteen amino acids
7. water soluble, fat soluble
8. a. vitamin C, b. vitamin K, c. vitamin B_{12}, d. vitamin D, e. riboflavin, f. vitamin A, g. vitamin E, h. pyridoxine (B_6)
9. a. iron; b. potassium; c. calcium; d. iodine; e. calcium, phosphorus, and fluorine; f. magnesium and sodium; g. chlorine; h. zinc
10. digestion of food, makes up blood plasma, helps tissues absorb nutrients, moves waste material; six to eight glasses
11. digestion breaks down food into smaller parts and changes food chemically, absorption is the process where blood capillaries pick up digested nutrients
12. kilocalorie (or calorie)
13. (Any 4 of the following) activity, age, size, sex, physical condition, climate
14. activity, caloric intake
15. Calculation of calories will vary with student weight: weight should be multiplied by 15; 500; student subtracts 500 from daily calories; 500; student adds 500 to daily calories
16. answers will be individualized; students should explain why they think a religious dietary restriction could be detrimental to good nutrition
17. answers will be individualized; ascertain that students have calculated their weight correctly based on height
18. measures weight in relation to height and correlates this with body fat; calculation of BMI will be individualized but ascertain that student's graphic reading is accurate
19. underweight, overweight, obese
20. (Any 3 of the following) student must explain the importance of the guidelines chosen: balance calories from food and beverages with calories expended; prevent gradual weight gain; engage in at least 30 minutes of moderate-intensity physical activity most days of the week; consume less than 10 percent of calories from saturated fatty acids and less than 30 milligrams of cholesterol daily; keep daily total fat intake to between 25 and 35 percent of calories consumed; select lean, low-fat foods whenever possible; eat more fiber-rich foods; limit foods high in sugar and salt

C. **Menu Plans:** Answers will be individualized. Make sure the requirements for a 2,000-calorie diet have been met: 3 cups milk and milk products, 2½ cups vegetables, 2 cups fruits, 6 ounces of grains, and 5½ ounces of meat and beans. A sample menu is shown.

Breakfast: fruit, cereal, milk

Lunch: fruit, meat/fish/poultry/beans, vegetable, 2 bread, milk

Dinner: salad, meat/fish/poultry/beans, vegetable, rice/potato/pasta, milk, dessert

Snacks: raw vegetables, fruit, crackers, cereal

D. **Therapeutic Diets:** Students may list any four of the foods for each diet.

1. Soft: meat and shellfish with tough connective tissue, coarse cereals, spicy foods, rich desserts, fried foods, raw fruits and vegetables, nuts, coconut
2. Diabetic: candy, soft drinks, desserts, cookies, syrup, honey, condensed milk, chewing gum, jams and jellies
3. Low-calorie: butter, cream, whole milk, cream soups and gravies, sweet soft drinks, alcohol, salad dressings, fatty meats, candy, rich desserts
4. High-calorie: green salads, watermelon, fibrous fruits, fried foods, rich pastries, cheesecake
5. Low-cholesterol: beef, liver, pork, lamb, egg yolk, cream cheese, natural cheeses, whole milk, coconut and palm oil products, shellfish
6. Fat-restricted: cream, whole milk, cheese, fats, fatty meats, rich desserts, chocolate, fried foods, salad dressings, nuts, coconut
7. Sodium-restricted: salt added to food, smoked meats/fish, processed foods, pickles, sauerkraut, processed cheese, olives
8. Low-protein: meats, fish, milk, cheese, eggs
9. Bland: coarse foods, fried foods, highly seasoned foods, pastries, candies, raw fruits and vegetables, alcoholic and carbonated beverages, smoked and salted meats/fish, nuts, olives, avocados, coconut, whole grain breads and cereals, coffee, tea
10. Low-residue: raw fruits and vegetables, whole grain breads and cereals, nuts, seeds, beans, peas, coconut, fried foods

CHAPTER 12 COMPUTER TECHNOLOGY IN HEALTH CARE

1. information systems, diagnostic testing, educational tools, research
2. ability to understand the basics of how the computer works and applications used in a field or profession
3. (Any 8 of the following) watches, cameras, telephones, thermometers, blood pressure gauges, cars, satellite navigation equipment, stoves, burglar alarm systems, personal computers
4. electronic, information processing center, calculate, store, sort, update, manipulate, sequence, organize, process
5. hardware is the components of the machine, and software is the programs or instructions that run the hardware
6. (Any 6 of the following) keypad, keyboard, mouse, optical scanner, light pen, bar code reader, card reader, disk, tape, CD-ROM, videodisc, touch screen, voice, microphone, DVD
7. processes all information or data entering the computer, acts as "brains" of the computer
8. read-only memory is permanent memory built and stored in the computer system by the manufacturer; random-access memory is not permanent because data can be stored, changed, and/or retrieved
9. finished work of a computer; printer, video display monitor
10. (Any 5 of the following) word processing documents, compiling databases, scheduling, maintaining financial records, monitoring patients, performing diagnostic tests, maintaining inventories, developing spreadsheets, communicating through modems
11. use access codes or special passwords to limit access to the information

12. allows physician to see cross-sectional views of bone and body tissues; regular X-rays show little depth, and soft tissue does not appear clearly
13. uses high-frequency sound waves that bounce back as an echo when they hit different tissues and organs
14. networks, communication
15. process of creating and sending messages from one computer to another
16. (Any 3 of the following) files created in word processing programs, insurance forms, financial data, X-rays or radiographic images, photographs
17. a. telemedicine
    b. telepharmacies
    c. e-medicine
18. organ transplant work
19. computer, modem, service provider, browser
20. a. CAI: computer-assisted instruction
    b. CPU: central processing unit
    c. CRT: cathode ray tube
    d. CT: computerized tomography
    e. HIS: hospital information system
    f. MIS: medical information system
    g. MRI: magnetic resonance imaging
    h. PET: positron emission tomography
    i. RAM: random-access memory
    j. ROM: read-only memory
21. electrical surges, power outages, viruses, hackers
22. through downloading of information from the Internet, through opening of contaminated e-mails, through use of disks or tapes that contain viruses
23. a protective program that limits the ability of other computers to access a computer
24. (Any 4 of the following) keep passwords confidential, prevent others from watching while keying a password, do not allow others to read the computer screen, clear the monitor before leaving the area, never open or download files or e-mails from an unknown party, follow the instructions if a virus or firewall alert occurs, shred discarded hard copies and printouts

CHAPTER 13 PROMOTION OF SAFETY

CHAPTER 13:1 USING BODY MECHANICS

1. way in which the body moves and maintains balance by the most efficient use of all of its parts
2. (Any 4 of the following) muscles work best when used correctly; correct use of muscles makes pushing, pulling, and lifting easier; prevents unnecessary fatigue and strain; saves energy; prevents injury to self and others
3. Diagram 1: maintain broad base of support, use strongest muscles, use weight of your body to help push

   Diagram 2: maintain broad base of support, use strongest muscles, stand close and carry heavy objects close to body

   Diagram 3: maintain broad base of support, bend from hips and knees, use strongest muscles

CHAPTER 13:2 PREVENTING ACCIDENTS AND INJURIES

1. Occupational Safety & Health Administration, establish and enforce standards for the workplace
2. (Any 4 of the following) product identification information, protection or precautions that must be used; instructions for safe use; procedures for handling spills, cleanup, and disposal; emergency first aid procedures
3. sodium hypochlorite
4. (Any 6 of the following) blood, blood components, urine, stool, semen, vaginal secretions, cerebrospinal fluid, saliva, mucus
5. hepatitis B, hepatitis C, and acquired immunodeficiency syndrome (AIDS)

6. (Any 5 of the following) read Material Safety Data Sheets (MSDSs) before using any hazardous chemical solutions; make sure all solution bottles are labeled; read the labels at least three times to make sure you have the correct solution; do not mix any solutions together unless instructed to do so by the instructor or immediate supervisor; some solutions can be poisonous—avoid contact with your eyes and skin; avoid inhaling any fumes displaced by a solution; store all chemical solutions in a locked cabinet or closet; dispose of solutions according to instructions provided on the MSDS; if you spill any solutions, immediately report the incident to the instructor or immediate supervisor
7. (Any 4 of the following) keep equipment in proper location at all times; dry your hands thoroughly before handling any electrical equipment; do not operate any equipment until you have been instructed on how to use it; read and follow the operating instructions for all major pieces of equipment; do not operate any equipment if your instructor is not in the room; report any damaged or malfunctioning equipment immediately; do not use frayed or damaged electrical cords; if you break any equipment, immediately report the incident to the instructor or immediate supervisor; observe all safety precautions when handling any equipment
8. (Any 4 of the following) do not perform any procedure unless you have been instructed to do so; provide privacy for all patients; identify your patient; explain the procedure to the patient; never perform a procedure on a patient if he or she refuses to allow you to do it; observe the patient closely during any procedure; check the area frequently for safety hazards; observe all safety checkpoints before leaving a patient
9. (Any 2 of the following) knock on door, speak to the patient and identify yourself before going behind privacy curtains, close door and/or draw curtains before beginning a procedure
10. (Any 2 of the following) check identification wrist band, ask the patient to state his or her name, repeat name twice, check name on record or bed
11. (Any 5 of the following) leave patient in comfortable position, elevate siderails if indicated, lower bed to lowest level, lock the bed wheels, place the call signal in reach, open privacy curtains, leave area neat and clean
12. before and after any procedure, anytime they become contaminated
13. when instructed to do so and in situations that might result in possible eye injury
14. a. report the cut to the instructor immediately; b. inform the instructor; do not attempt to remove the particle or rub the eye; c. report the malfunctioning equipment immediately; d. report the spilled acid to the instructor; e. do not use the cord; report it immediately

CHAPTER 13:3 OBSERVING FIRE SAFETY

1. oxygen, fuel, and heat
2. (Any 4 of the following) smoking and matches, misuse of electricity, defects in heating systems, spontaneous ignition, improper rubbish disposal, arson
3. (Any 3 of the following) obey all No Smoking signs; extinguish matches and cigarettes completely; dispose of all waste materials in correct containers; check all electrical equipment for damaged cords or improper grounding; store flammable materials in proper containers, do not allow clutter to accumulate; observe special precautions when oxygen is in use
4. Answer depends on school's location
5. Answers depend on location and kind of extinguisher
6.

Class	Uses on what type of fires?
A	Combustibles paper, cloth, plastic, wood
B	Flammable or combustible liquids Gasoline, oil, paints, grease cooking fat
C	Electrical Fuse boxes, appliances, wiring, electrical outlets
D	Burning or combustile metals

7. a. Class A; b. Class C; c. Class A, B, and C; d. Class B and C
8. carbon dioxide and dry chemical
9. R: rescue anyone in immediate danger
   A: activate the alarm
   C: contain the fire
   E: extinguish the fire or evacuate the area
10. (Any 3 of the following) post "No Smoking—Oxygen in Use" sign; remove all smoking materials, candles, lighters, and matches from the room; avoid use of electrically operated equipment; do not use flammable liquids; avoid static electricity
11. stay calm, follow the policy of the health care facility, provide for the safety of yourself and the patient
12. legally

CHAPTER 13 SAFETY EXAMINATION

1. A	7. B	13. D	19. True	25. False
2. B	8. C	14. True	20. True	26. False
3. A	9. A	15. False	21. False	27. True
4. A	10. B	16. True	22. False	28. True
5. D	11. A	17. True	23. True	29. False
6. C	12. C	18. True	24. True	30. True

31. a. Class A — Combustibles: paper, cloth, plastic, wood
    b. Class B — Flammable or combustible liquids: gasoline, oil, paints, grease, fats
    c. Class C — Electrical: fuse boxes, appliances, wiring, electrical outlets
    d. Class D — Burning or combustible metals
32. (Any 3 rules for preventing fires are acceptable) obey all "No Smoking" signs, extinguish matches and cigarettes, dispose of waste materials in correct containers, check all electrical equipment before use, store flammable materials in proper containers, do not allow clutter to accumulate
33. Occupational Health & Safety Administration; to establish and enforce standards for the workplace
34. check Material Safety Data Sheet (MSDS)
35. hepatitis B, hepatitis C, and acquired immunodeficiency syndrome (AIDS)

CHAPTER 14 INFECTION CONTROL

CHAPTER 14:1 UNDERSTANDING THE PRINCIPLES OF INFECTION CONTROL

1. Answers to crossword puzzle

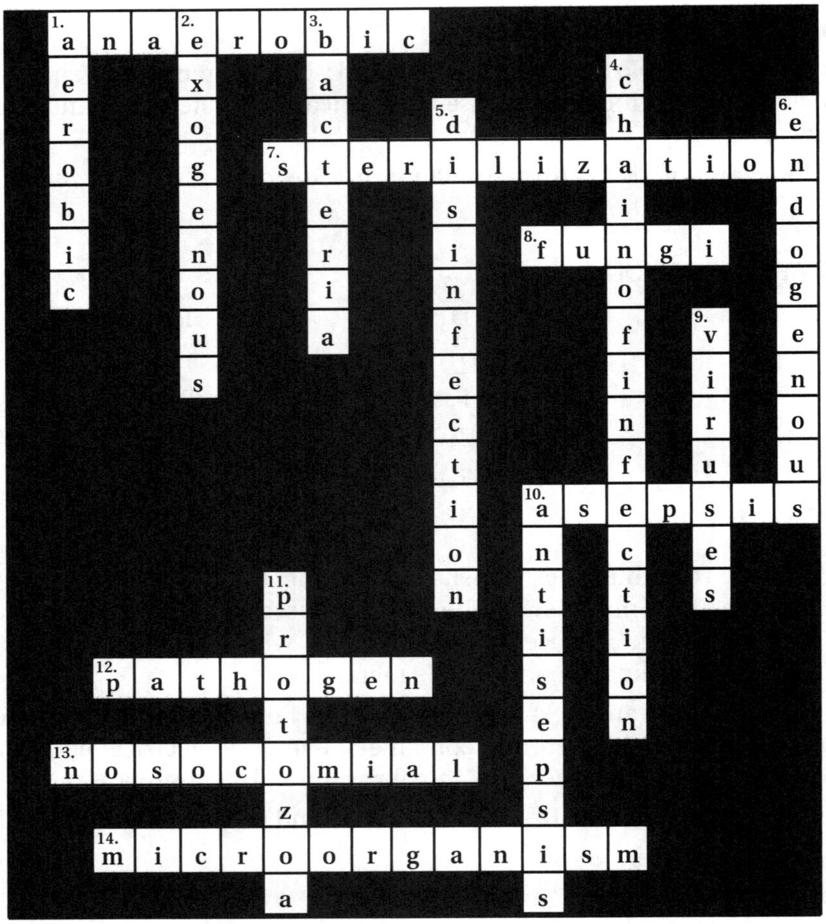

2. nonpathogens are microorganisms that are beneficial in maintaining certain body processes; pathogens are microorganisms that cause infection and disease
3. a. bacilli
   b. vibrio
   c. streptococci
   d. spirilla
   e. staphylococci
4. a. viruses, b. rickettsiae, c. protozoa, d. fungi, e. rickettsiae, f. bacteria, g. viruses, h. fungi
5. a. West Nile virus (WNV)
   b. H5N1 virus
   c. severe acute respiratory syndrome (SARS) virus
   d. Monkeypox hantavirus
   e. filoviruses such as Ebola and Marburg
   f. human immunodeficiency virus (HIV)
   g. hepatitis B (HBV) and hepatitis C (HCV)
6. must provide vaccination at no cost to any worker with exposure to blood or body secretions
7. (Any 3 of the following) warm environment, darkness, source of food and moisture, some need oxygen
8. (Any 2 of the following) produce poisons called toxins, cause allergic reaction, attack and destroy living cells
9. endogenous originates within the body, exogenous originates outside the body

10. staphylococcus, pseudomonas, and enterococci
11. establish infection control programs
12. a. mode of transmission and portal of exit
    b. portal of entry
    c. susceptible host
    d. reservoir or source and mode of transmission
    e. mode of transmission and source or reservoir
    f. causative agent
13. (Any 4 of the following) handwashing, good personal hygiene, using disposable gloves, proper cleaning of instruments and equipment, thorough cleaning of the environment
14. a. antisepsis: prevent or inhibit growth of pathogenic organisms but not effective against spores and viruses
    b. disinfection: destroys or kills pathogenic organisms but not always effective against spores and viruses
    c. sterilization: destroys all microorganisms, both pathogenic and nonpathogenic, including spores and viruses

CHAPTER 14:2 BIOTERRORISM

A. Matching

1. D	5. F	9. A	13. A
2. C	6. C	10. D	14. C
3. A	7. E	11. B	
4. B	8. F	12. E	

B. Competion and Short Answer

1. use of microorganisms or biologic agents as weapons to infect humans, animals, or plants
2. (Any 6 of the following) inexpensive and readily available; spread through air or contaminated food and water; survives sunlight, drying, and heat; causes death or severe disability; easily transmitted; difficult to prevent and/or treat
3. development of a comprehensive plan against bioterrorism
4. military, first responders, police, fire department and health care personnel; answers will be individualized but student should explain why this is important
5. so information can be transmitted quickly and efficiently
6. answers will be individualized; make sure student states why health care workers are or are not prepared

CHAPTER 14:3 WASHING HANDS

1. method followed to prevent the spread of germs or pathogens
2. washing hands prevents spread of pathogens from one person to another, protects health worker from disease and illness
3. (Any 6 of the following) when you arrive and immediately before leaving facility; before and after patient contact; any time hands become contaminated; before applying and immediately after removing gloves; before and after handling any specimen; after contact with soiled or contaminated linen; after picking up any item from the floor; after personal use of the bathroom; after you cough, sneeze, or use a tissue; before and after any contact with your mouth or mucous membrane
4. aids in removal of germs
5. fingers are pointed downward to prevent flow of water up forearm
6. warm water is used; hot water damages skin and cold does not create good lather
7. prevents contamination of hands from germs on faucet
8. palms, top or back of hands, between fingers
9. brush or blunt edge of orange stick
10. long or artificial nails can harbor organisms, increase the spread of infection, and puncture or tear gloves

11. a. antiseptic hand rub or waterless handwashing
    b. antiseptic handwashing using an antimicrobial soap and water
    c. regular handwashing using plain soap and water
    d. antiseptic handwashing using an antimicrobial soap and water
12. alcohol to provide antisepsis and a moisturizer to prevent drying of the skin
13. until they are dry, usually at least 15 seconds
14. six to ten times

CHAPTER 14:4 OBSERVING STANDARD PRECAUTIONS

1. hepatitis B virus, hepatitis C virus, human immunodeficient virus
2. Occupational Safety & Health Administration (OSHA)
3. (Any 4 of the following) gloves, gowns, lab coats, masks, face shields
4. no; federal law prohibits eating and drinking in any area potentially contaminated by blood or body fluids
5. provide a confidential medical evaluation and follow-up
6. identify and use effective and safe medical devices, incorporate changes in annual update of Exposure Control Plan, solicit input from nonmanagerial employees who are responsible for direct patient care, maintain a sharp's injury log
7. in any situation where health care provider might contact blood, body fluids, secretions, excretions, mucous membranes, nonintact skin, and/or tissue or cell specimens
8. whenever contact with blood, body fluids, secretions, excretions, mucous membranes, or nonintact skin is possible; handling any contaminated items or surfaces; performing invasive procedures; performing venipuncture or blood tests
9. during any procedure likely to cause splashing of blood, body fluids, secretions, or excretions
10. (Any 3 of the following) irrigation of wounds, suctioning, dental procedures, delivery of a baby, surgical procedures
11. every 30 minutes or anytime they become moist or wet
12. left uncapped and placed in leakproof, puncture-resistant sharps container
13. put on gloves, wipe area with disposable cleaning cloths and a disinfectant solution
14. avoid need for mouth-to-mouth resuscitation
15. infectious waste or biohazard material bag
16. report it immediately

CHAPTER 14:5 STERILIZING WITH AN AUTOCLAVE

1. steam, pressure, gas, microorganisms, pathogenic, nonpathogenic, spores, viruses
2. prepared properly, washed thoroughly and rinsed
3. (Any 3 of the following) muslin, autoclave paper, special plastic or paper bags, autoclave containers
4. to ensure that an article has been sterilized
5. (Any 2 of the following) tape, sensitive marks, capsules
6. (Any 3 of the following) space between all pieces; packages placed on side, not flat; jars, basins, and cans placed on sides; no articles in contact with side, door, or top of the autoclave
7. different articles require different pressure, temperature, and/or time
8. check directions provided with autoclave
9. wet surfaces permit rapid infiltration of organisms
10. clean, dustproof areas
11. 30 days
12. rewrap and autoclave the item
13. 320° to 350° F (160° to 177° C); 60 minutes
14. instruments that corrode, items destroyed by moisture

CHAPTER 14:6 USING CHEMICALS FOR DISINFECTION

1. spores, viruses, chemical disinfection, sterilization
2. (Any 3 of the following) instruments that do not penetrate body tissue, dental instruments, percussion hammers, scissors, thermometers
3. (Any 2 of the following) particles or debris contaminate chemical, soap reduces effectiveness, water dilutes
4. (Any 5 of the following) 90 percent isopropyl alcohol, formaldehyde-alcohol, 2 percent phenolic germicide, Lysol, Zephiran, benzalkonium, 10 percent bleach solution, Cidex, glutaraldehyde, iodophor
5. some must be diluted or mixed, obtain recommended time
6. prevent formation of rust; no; can cause a chemical reaction with some solutions and reduce effectiveness
7. ensures that all parts of article are disinfected
8. tight-fitting lid
9. drawer or dustfree closet
10. some after one use, any time contamination occurs or dirt is present, follow manufacturer's instructions

CHAPTER 14:7 CLEANING WITH AN ULTRASONIC UNIT

1. sound
2. bubbles strike article being cleaned, explode, and drive solution onto the article
3. no; does not remove spores or viruses
4. some solutions must be diluted, some can only be used on specific materials
5. toxic, can cause skin irritation
6. general all-purpose cleanser
7. bottoms should be below level of solution in the permanent tank
8. brush off most of the dirt or particles
9. pearls, pasted stones
10. discard and replace
11. drain by side valve, wipe with damp cloth or disinfectant
12. check cleaning chart

CHAPTER 14:8 USING STERILE TECHNIQUES

1. sterile: free from all organisms, including spores and viruses; contaminated: organisms and pathogens are present
2. hold out in front of body and above waist
3. two-inch border around the sterile field
4. drop: drop from wrapper onto sterile field; mitten: loose ends grasped to form mitten for handling; transfer forceps: use to grasp article and place on sterile field
5. organisms and pathogens travel quickly through a wet surface
6. discard and start over
7. inside (side against skin)
8. sterile tray is open and you are ready to do procedure
9. away from body and above waist
10. start over

CHAPTER 14:9 MAINTAINING TRANSMISSION-BASED ISOLATION PRECAUTIONS

1. method or technique of caring for patients who have communicable disease
2. an epidemic affects a large number of people at the same time, but a pandemic affects a wide geographic area and most of the population
3. standard precautions are used on all patients, transmission-based isolation techniques provide extra protection against specific diseases or pathogens to prevent their spread
4. disease caused by a pathogenic organism that can be easily transmitted to others

5. direct contact with patients; contact with dirty linen, equipment, and/or supplies; contact with blood, body fluids, secretions, and excretions
6. causative agent, way organism is transmitted, whether pathogen is antibiotic-resistant
7. contaminated: items that contain disease-producing organisms
8. clean: items that do not contain the disease-producing organisms and have minimal chance of spreading the disease
9. (1) A
   (2) C
   (3) D
   (4) B
   (5) A, B, C, D
   (6) B
   (7) A
   (8) C
   (9) A
   (10) B
   (11) A, B, C
   (12) C
   (13) A
   (14) A, B, C
10. method used to protect patients from organisms in environment
11. (Any 2 of the following) depressed immune system, severely burned, patients receiving chemotherapy or radiation treatment, immune system failed
12. (Any 4 of the following) room cleaned and disinfected; wear clean or sterile gowns, gloves, and masks; equipment and supplies are clean, disinfected, or sterile; filters are used to purify air

CHAPTER 15 VITAL SIGNS

CHAPTER 15:1 MEASURING AND RECORDING VITAL SIGNS

1. Answers to crossword puzzle

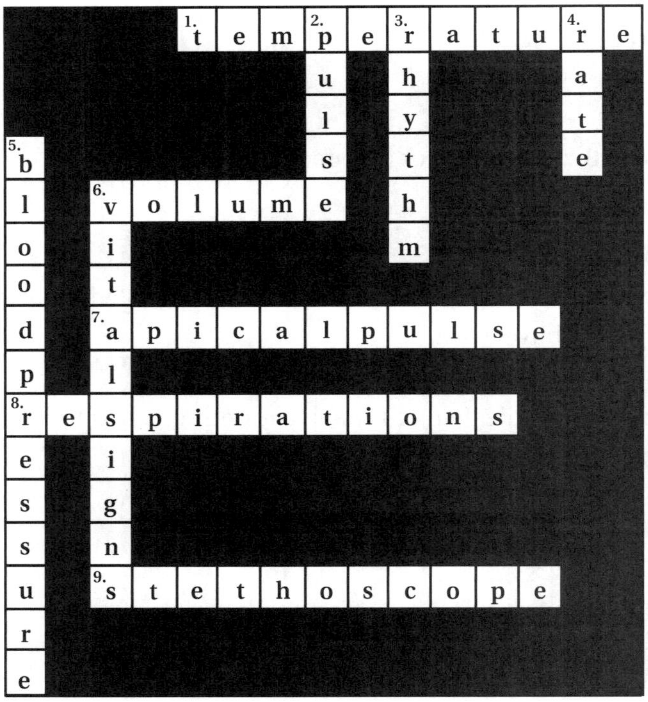

2. temperature, pulse, respiration, and blood pressure
3. often the first indication of a disease or an abnormality
4. orally, rectally, axillary, aurally
5. pressure of the blood felt against the wall of an artery as the heart contracts (or beats); rate, rhythm, volume
6. count or rate, rhythm, character
7. systolic, diastolic
8. (Any 3 of the following) illness, hardening of the arteries, weak or rapid radial pulse, doctor's order, infants and children

9. report it to your supervisor immediately
10. ask another individual to check the patient
11. a. 60° C
    b. 21.1° C
    c. 10° C
    d. 3.3° C
    e. 30° C
    f. 40.6° C
    g. 58.9° C
    h. 95.6° C
    i. 37.6° C
    j. –3.9° C
12. a. 89.6° F
    b. 129.2° F
    c. 46.4° F
    d. 195.8° F
    e. 32° F
    f. 161.6° F
    g. 78.8° F
    h. 177.8° F
    i. 211.6° F
    j. 115° F

CHAPTER 15:2 MEASURING AND RECORDING TEMPERATURE

1. balance between heat lost and heat produced in the body
2. individual differences, time of day, parts of the body
3. 97–100° F, or 36.1–37.8° C
4. 98.6° F, or 37° C, 3–5 minutes
5. 99.6° F, or 37.6° C, 3–5 minutes
6. 97.6° F, or 36.4° C, 10 minutes
7. rectal or temporal: internal temperature; it measures the temperature inside the body
8. axillary or groin; external temperature
9. temperature recorded in ear or auditory canal
10. measures thermal infrared energy radiating from tympanic membrane, or eardrum
11. measures the blood temperature in the temporal artery
12. hypothermia is low body temperature below 95° F (35° C), hyperthermia is high body temperature above 104° F (40° C)
13. short, stubby, rounded bulb; red tip
14. put on gloves, use two cards to push droplets of mercury and glass into a plastic container with a tight fitting lid, wipe area with damp sponge, put all cleanup material into plastic container, label "Mercury for recycling," and take tightly sealed container to mercury recycling center
15. place disposable cover over probe
16. special chemical dots or strips change color when exposed to specific temperatures
17. eating, drinking, or smoking can alter temperature in mouth
18. 30 minutes
19. Reading a Thermometer

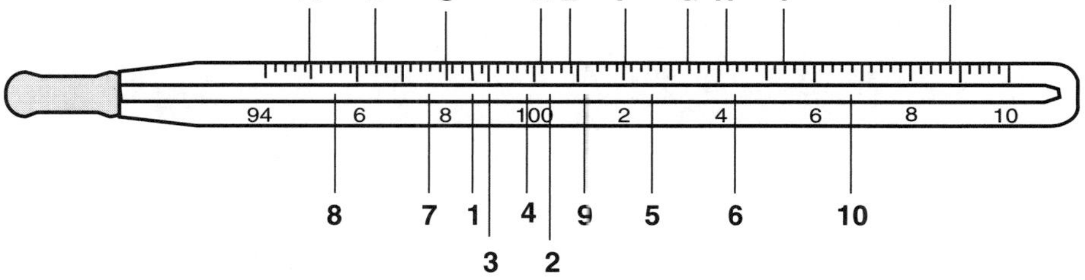

20. A. 95
    B. 96^4
    C. 98
    D. 100^2
    E. 100^8
    F. 102
    G. 103^4
    H. 104^2
    I. 105^4
    J. 108^8

CHAPTER 15:3 MEASURING AND RECORDING PULSE

1. pressure of the blood felt against the wall of an artery as the heart beats and rests
2. A. temporal
   B. carotid
   C. brachial
   D. radial
   E. femoral
   F. popliteal
   G. dorsalis pedis
   Part (b) Circle radial pulse (D)
3. rate, rhythm, volume
4. a. 60 to 100 b. 70 to 100 c. 80 to 110 d. 100 to 160
5. (Any 3 of the following) exercise, stimulant drugs, excitement, fever, shock, nervous tension
6. (Any 3 of the following) sleep, depressant drugs, heart disease, coma, physical training
7. bradycardia, tachycardia, arrhythmia

CHAPTER 15:4 MEASURING AND RECORDING RESPIRATIONS

1. the process involving taking in of oxygen and expelling of carbon dioxide by the lungs and respiratory tract
2. inspiration, expiration
3. adults: 12–20 per minute; children: 16–30 per minute; infants: 30–50 per minute
4. (Any 4 of the following) deep, shallow, labored, difficult, moist, stertorous
5. regular, irregular
6. a. dyspnea: difficult or labored respirations (breathing)
   b. apnea: absence of respirations, usually a temporary period of no respirations
   c. Cheyne–Stokes: abnormal breathing pattern characterized by periods of dyspnea followed by periods of apnea
   d. rales: bubbling or noisy sounds caused by fluids or mucus in the air passages
   e. tachypnea: respiratory rate above 25 respirations per minute
   f. bradypnea: respiratory rate below 10 respirations per minute
   g. wheezing: difficult breathing with high-pitched whistling or sighing sounds during expiration
   h. cyanosis: a dusky, bluish discoloration of the skin, lips, and/or nail beds as a result of decreased oxygen and increased carbon dioxide in the bloodstream
7. if patient is aware, he or she can alter the rate of breathing
8. leave hand in position on radial pulse, but count respirations

CHAPTER 15:5 ASSIGNMENT SHEETS #1–5 GRAPHING

Assignment Sheet #1 **15:5 Graphing TPR**

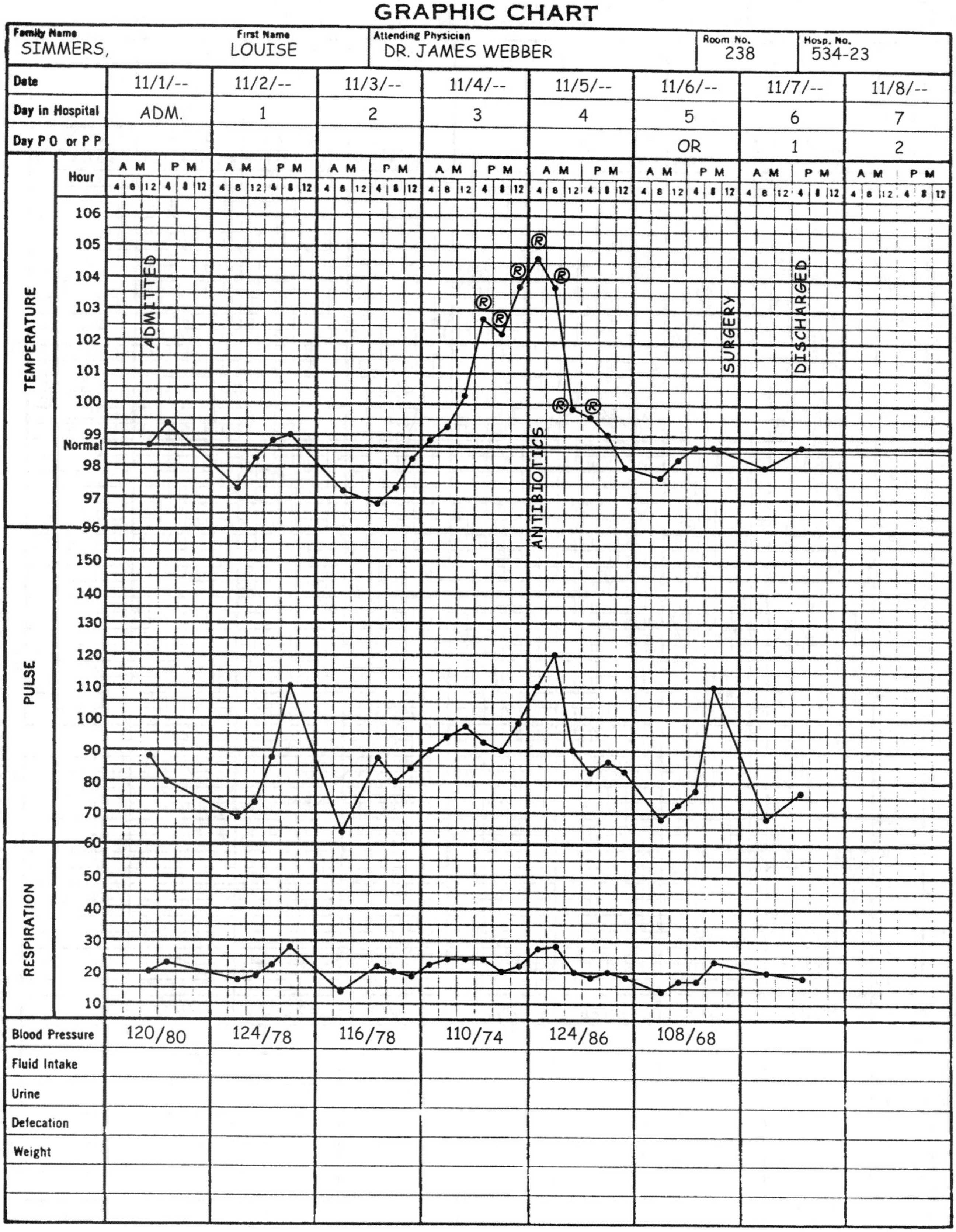

Assignment Sheet #2 **15:5 Graphing TPR**

GRAPHIC CHART

Family Name	First Name	Attending Physician	Room No.	Hosp. No.
PETRO	TAMIKA	DR. JOHN VAUGHN	238	36-26-38

Date	11/8/--	11/9/--	11/10/--	11/11/--	11/12/--	11/13/--	11/14/--	11/15/--
Day in Hospital	ADM.	1	2	3	4	5	6	7
Day P O or P P		OR	1	2	3	4	5	6

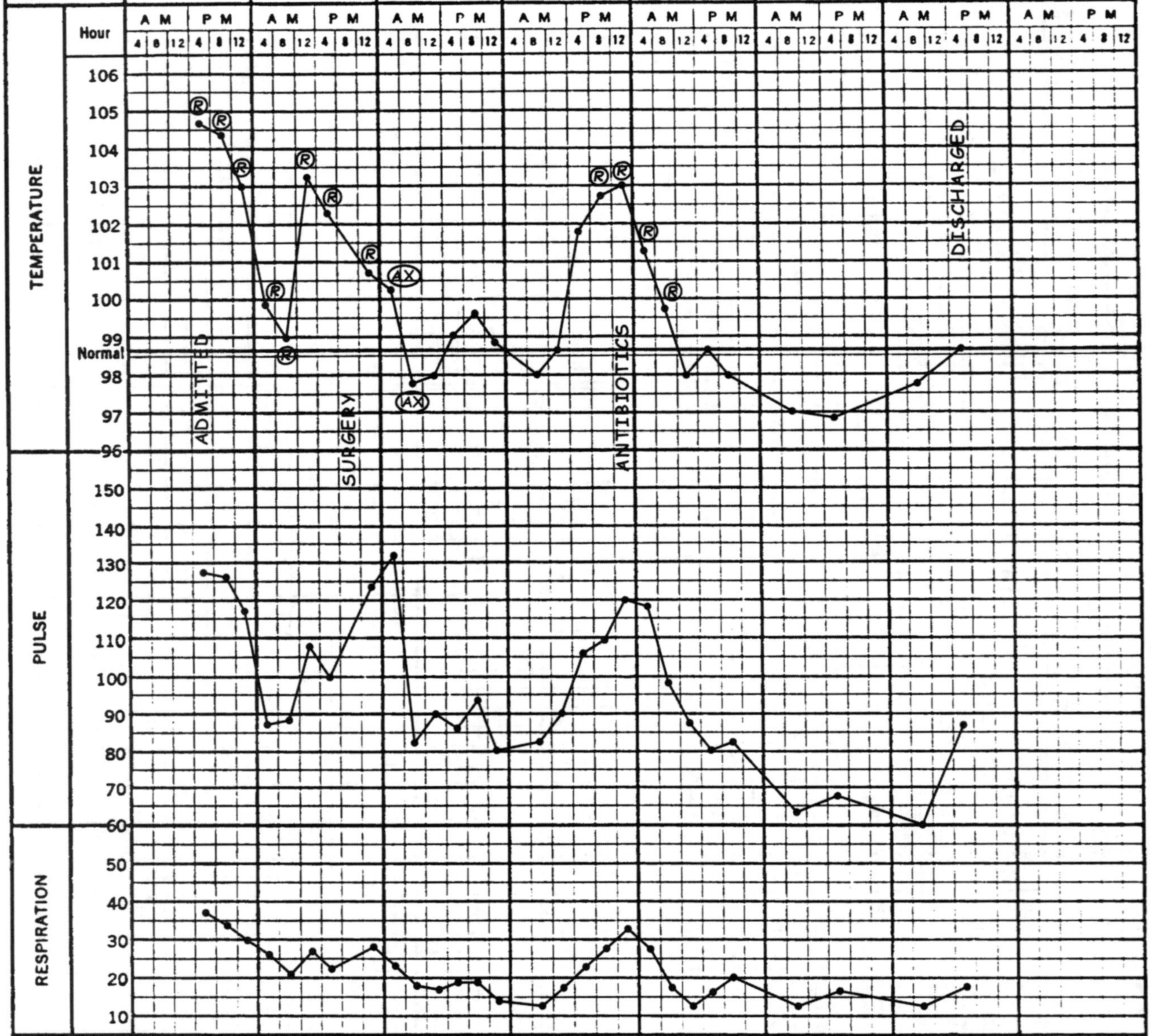

Blood Pressure	134/86	124/76	110/68	106/68	108/78	122/82	120/78	
Fluid Intake								
Urine								
Defecation								
Weight								

Assignment Sheet #3 **15:5 Graphing TPR**

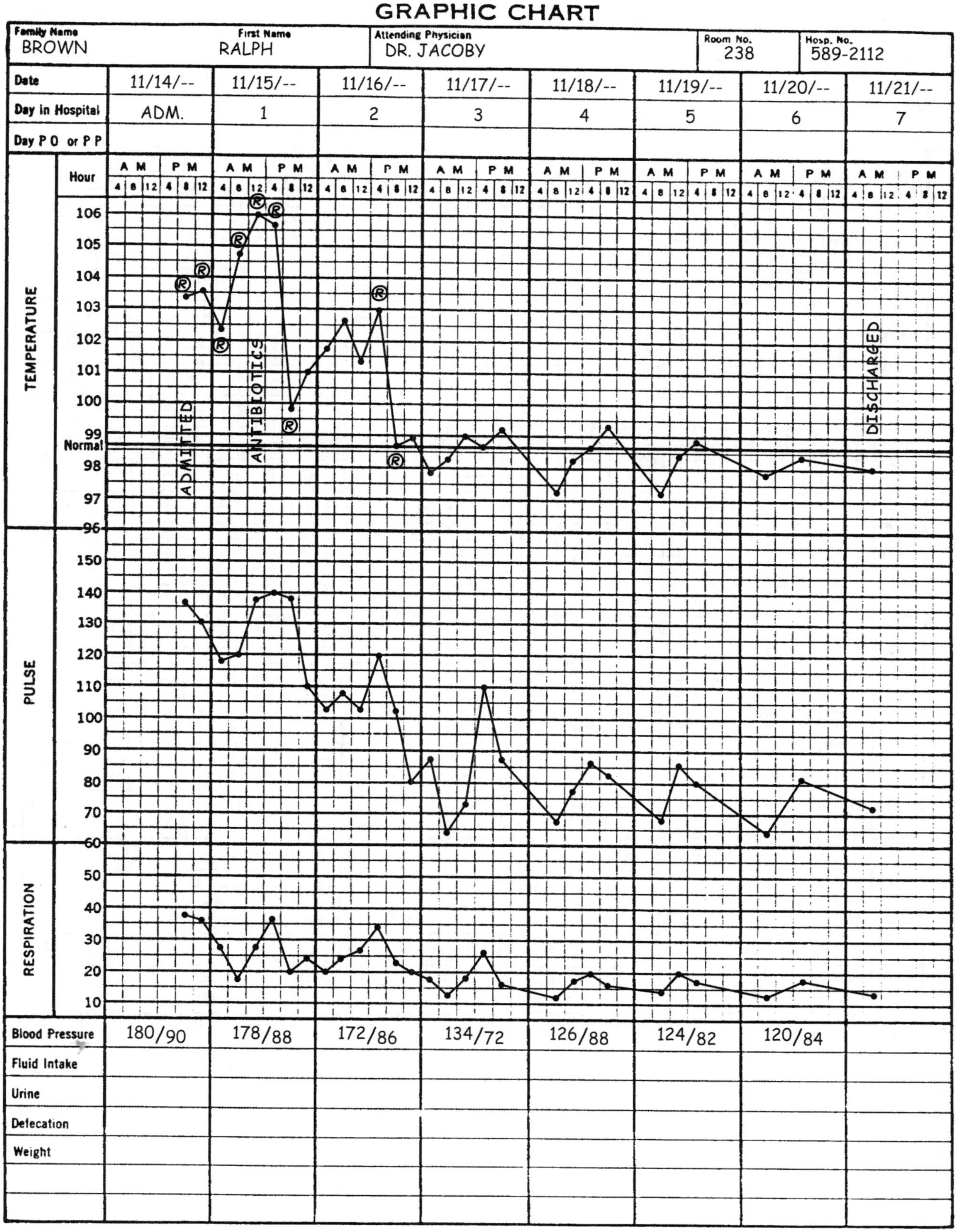

Assignment Sheet #4 — **15:5 Graphing TPR**

GRAPHIC CHART

Family Name	First Name	Attending Physician	Room No.	Hosp. No.
DAUGHERTY	ROGER	DR. YODER	238	555-44

Date	11/28/--	11/29/--	11/30/--	12/1/--	12/2/--	12/3/--	12/4/--	12/5/--
Day in Hospital	ADM.	1	2	3	4	5	6	7
Day P O or P P								

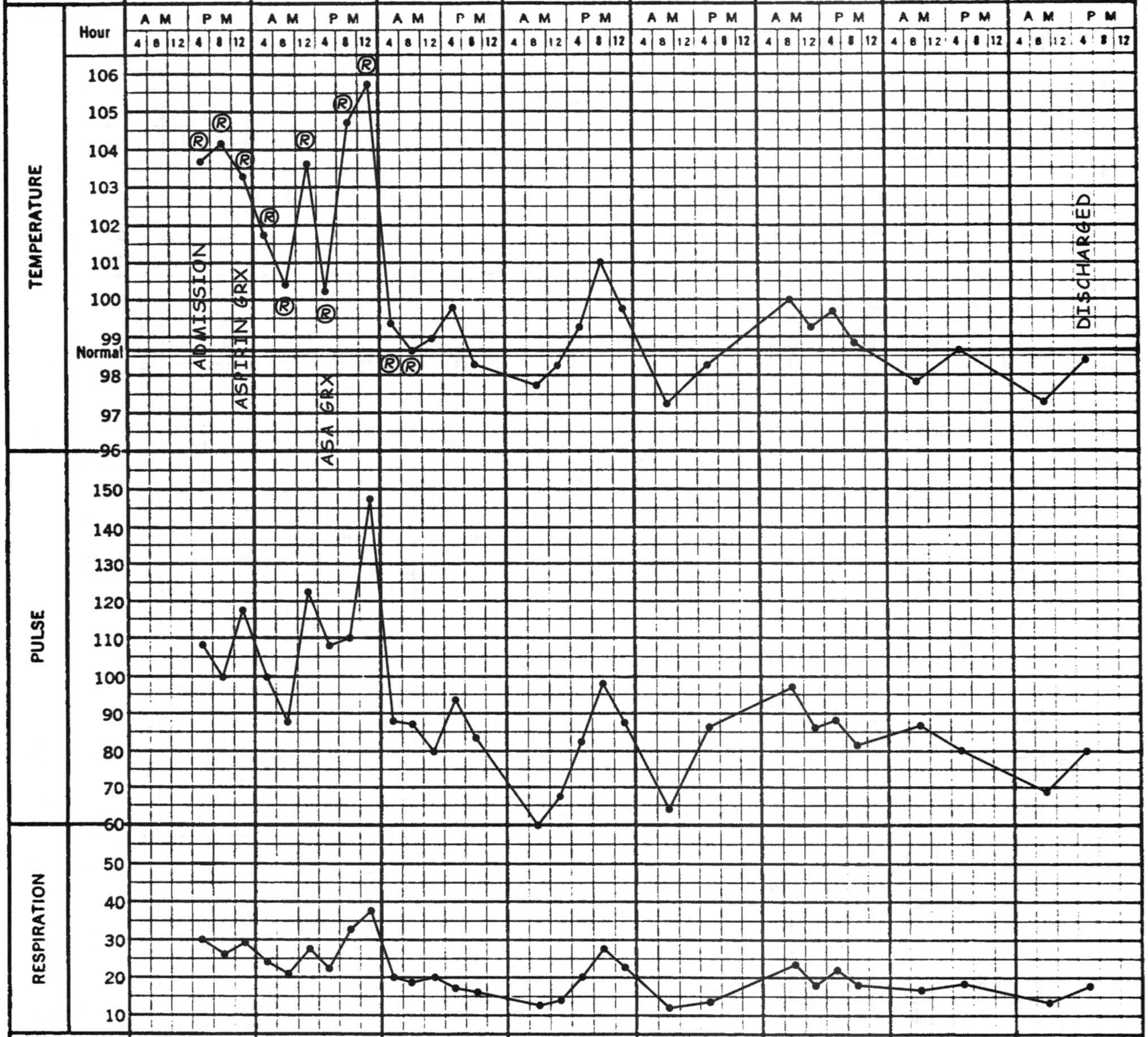

Blood Pressure	128/80	124/84	118/76	130/78	126/76	114/76	118/78	118/76
Fluid Intake								
Urine								
Defecation								
Weight	200							

Assignment Sheet #5 **15:5 Graphing TPR**

GRAPHIC CHART

Family Name	First Name	Attending Physician	Room No.	Hosp. No.
JOHNSON	JIM	DR. IMHOFF	238	54-56-54

Date	1/1/--	1/2/--	1/3/--	1/4/--	1/5/--	1/6/--	1/7/--	1/8/--
Day in Hospital	ADM.	1	2	3	4	5	6	7
Day P O or P P								

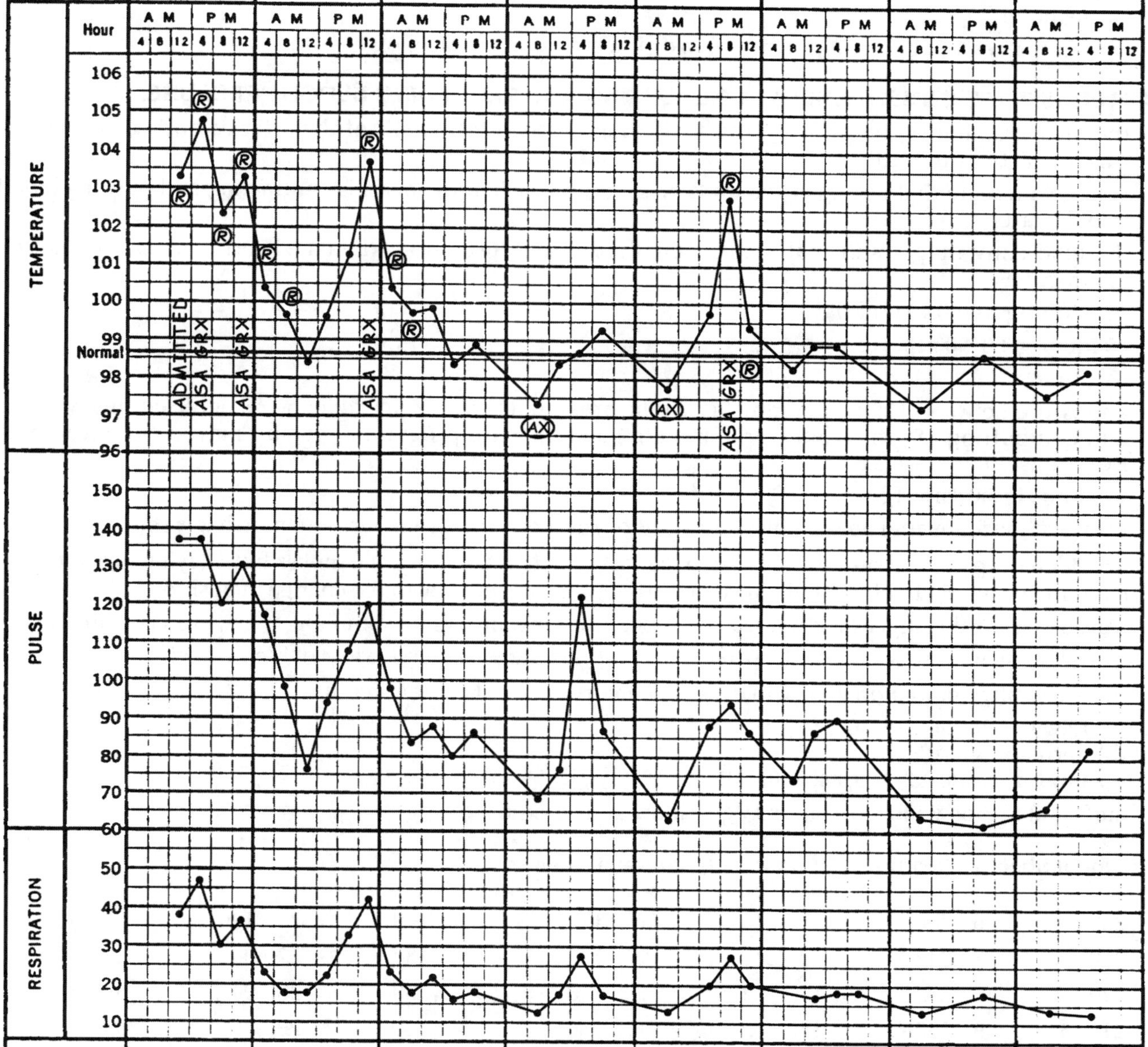

Blood Pressure	138/84	124/78	128/76	118/78	120/80	124/72	128/74	120/68
Fluid Intake								
Urine								
Defecation								
Weight	206							

CHAPTER 15:6 MEASURING AND RECORDING APICAL PULSE

1. a pulse count taken at the apex of the heart with a stethoscope
2. (Any 2 of the following) irregular heartbeats, hardening of the arteries, weak radial pulse, rapid radial pulse
3. infants and children have very rapid radial pulses
4. sounds are caused by the closing of the heart valves as blood flows through the chambers of the heart
5. report to your supervisor immediately
6. heart contractions are not strong enough to produce a pulse sensation at the radial site
7. 24, 46, none
8. wipe earpieces and bell/diaphragm with a disinfectant such as alcohol

CHAPTER 15:7 ASSIGNMENT SHEET #1 MEASURING AND RECORDING BLOOD PRESSURE

1. the measurement of the pressure that the blood exerts on the walls of the arteries during the various stages of activity in the heart
2. systolic: pressure that occurs in the walls of the arteries when the heart is contracting and pushing blood into the arteries
3. diastolic: constant pressure that is present in the walls of the arteries when the heart is at rest, or between contractions
4. 120 mm Hg, 100–140 mm Hg
5. 80 mm Hg, 60–90 mm Hg
6. 64
7. a pressure between 120 to 139 mmHg systolic or 80 to 89 mmHg diastolic; by recognizing this warning and committing to proper nutrition and a regular exercise program, a person may avoid developing hypertension
8. 140 mm Hg, 90 mm Hg
9. (Any 3 of the following) heart failure, dehydration, depression, severe burns, hemorrhage, shock
10. a sudden drop in both systolic and diastolic pressure when an individual moves from a lying to a sitting or standing position; inability of blood vessels to compensate quickly to the change in position
11. (Any 3 of the following) excitement, anxiety, nervous tension, eating, stimulant drugs, exercise, smoking
12. (Any 3 of the following) rest or sleep, depressant drugs, shock, excessive loss of blood, fasting
13. mercury sphygmomanometers can cause a mercury spill and contamination
14. (a) 128/92, 188/84, 136/76, 210/118
    (b) normal: 136/76
    (c) abnormal: 128/92, 188/84, 210/118
15. cuffs that are too wide or too narrow give inaccurate readings

Assignment Sheet #2 Reading a Mercury Sphygmomanometer

1. 298	6. 258	11. 216	16. 176	21. 140	26. 106	31. 68
2. 288	7. 248	12. 210	17. 166	22. 132	27. 98	32. 60
3. 280	8. 242	13. 204	18. 160	23. 128	28. 94	33. 54
4. 274	9. 232	14. 192	19. 150	24. 120	29. 86	34. 48
5. 268	10. 226	15. 186	20. 146	25. 114	30. 74	35. 38

Assignment Sheet #3 Reading an Aneroid Sphygmomanometer

1. 20	6. 76	11. 116	16. 158	21. 208	26. 276
2. 34	7. 82	12. 130	17. 170	22. 222	
3. 42	8. 90	13. 134	18. 178	23. 236	
4. 52	9. 98	14. 142	19. 186	24. 244	
5. 62	10. 104	15. 150	20. 198	25. 260	

CHAPTER 16 FIRST AID

CHAPTER 16:1 PROVIDING FIRST AID

1. the immediate care that is given to the victim of an accident or illness to minimize the effect of the injury or illness until experts can take over
2. life, death, recovery, permanent disability
3. (Any 3 of the following) type of injury or illness, environment, others present, equipment or supplies available, availability of medical help
4. (Any 3 of the following) listen for unusual sounds, look for unusual sights, note any odors, watch for unusual appearance or behavior
5. call for medical help and allow professionals to take over
6. whether victim is conscious
7. victim can be injured more severely by improper movement
8. (Any 5 of the following) situation, actions taken, exact location, telephone number, assistance required, number of people involved, condition of victim(s)
9. do not proceed with care; if possible, have someone witness refusal of care; call EMS and allow professionals to take over if a life-threatening emergency exists
10. method of prioritizing treatment
11. (Any 6 of the following) no breathing; difficult breathing; no pulse; severe bleeding; persistent pain in the chest or abdomen; vomiting or passing blood; poisoning; head, neck, or spine injuries; open chest or abdominal wounds; shock; severe partial-thickness and all full-thickness burns
12. (Any 4 of the following) victim, others present, items noted at scene, emergency medical identification, empty medicine containers, bottles of chemicals or solutions
13. present a confident, calm attitude
14. maintain confidentiality and protect victim's right to privacy
15. injury, qualified

CHAPTER 16:2 PERFORMING CARDIOPULMONARY RESUSCITATION (CPR)

1. cardiopulmonary resuscitation
2. A: airway; B: breathing; C: circulation, D: defibrillation
3. clinical death occurs when the heart stops beating and the victim stops breathing; biological death is death of cells
4. 4–6 minutes after clinical death
5. head tilt/chin lift method, jaw-thrust maneuver
6. automated external defibrillators, AED determines heart rhythms and sends audible or visual warning telling operator to push "shock" button
7. if any other rescuers are touching the victim when the shock is administered, they could receive severe injuries and even go into cardiac arrest
8. whether the victim is conscious
9. a. call fast, b. call first, c. call first, d. call fast, e. call fast
10. look, listen, feel
11. carotid
12. avoid pressure on the xiphoid process
13. 30, 2, 100, 5, $1\frac{1}{2}$ to 2, 3.8 to 5
14. 30:2
15. feel for a carotid pulse while chest compressions are administered
16. nose, mouth, lower half of the sternum, $\frac{1}{3}$ to $\frac{1}{2}$ of the depth of the chest, 100, 30, 2, 30:2
17. 100, lower half of the sternum, $\frac{1}{3}$ to $\frac{1}{2}$ the depth of the chest, 30:2
18. remain calm and encourage victim to cough hard
19. give 5 back blows, give 5 chest thrusts, check the mouth and sweep with a finger if the object is seen, attempt to ventilate
20. victim recovers, qualified help arrives, doctor orders you to discontinue attempt, rescuer becomes physically exhausted, scene becomes unsafe, you are given a legally valid do not resuscitate (DNR) order

CHAPTER 16:3 PROVIDING FIRST AID FOR BLEEDING AND WOUNDS

1. an open wound has a break in skin or mucous membrane and a closed wound does not
2. bleeding, infection
3. a. abrasion, b. incision, c. laceration, d. puncture, e. avulsion, f. amputation
4. a. spurts from wound, heavy blood loss, bright red in color; b. slower, steadier, dark red or maroon, constant but easier to control; c. oozes from wound, less red than arterial, clots easily
5. (1) direct pressure, (2) elevation, (3) pressure bandage, (4) pressure on pressure points
6. gloves, plastic wrap
7. brachial artery, femoral artery
8. (Any 4 of the following) wash hands, wear gloves, use sterile gauze with soap and water to wash wound, discard wipe after one use, wipe in outward direction when cleaning wound, apply sterile dressing or bandage
9. (Any 5 of the following) swelling, heat, redness, pain, fever, pus, red streaks leading from the wound
10. obtain medical advice regarding protection with tetanus shot
11. by a physician
12. (Any 6 of the following) pain; tenderness; swelling; deformity; cold, clammy skin; rapid weak pulse; a drop in blood pressure; uncontrolled restlessness; excessive thirst; vomited blood; blood in urine or feces
13. (Any 4 of the following) get medical help, check breathing, treat for shock, avoid unnecessary movement, avoid giving any fluids or food to the victim
14. shock
15. calm, medical

CHAPTER 16:4 PROVIDING FIRST AID FOR SHOCK

1. a clinical set of signs and various symptoms that are associated with an inadequate supply of blood to body organs
2. brain, heart
3. (Any 6 of the following) hemorrhage; excessive pain; infection; heart attack; stroke; poisoning by chemicals, drugs, or gases; lack of oxygen; psychological trauma; dehydration from burns, vomiting, or diarrhea
4. a. septic, b. cardiogenic, c. hemorrhagic, d. anaphylactic, e. psychogenic, f. metabolic
5. (Any 10 of the following) skin pale or cyanotic; skin cool; excessive perspiration (diaphoresis); wet, clammy skin; rapid, weak pulse; rapid, shallow respirations; irregular respirations; low blood pressure; weak; confused; loss of consciousness; anxiety and restlessness; excessive thirst; nausea and/or vomiting; blurred vision; sunken or vacant expression in eyes; dilated pupils
6. cause of shock, circulation, adequate oxygen, body temperature
7. a. neck or spine: do not move
   b. vomiting: lying on side
   c. respiratory distress: raise victim's head and shoulders
   d. none of previous present: lying flat with feet raised approximately 12 inches
8. remove some blankets to avoid overheating the victim

CHAPTER 16:5 PROVIDING FIRST AID FOR POISONING

1. ingestion (swallowing), inhalation, skin contact with harmful substances, injection (bite or sting)
2. type, injury, contact
3. on the side; so fluids can drain from the mouth
4. call poison control center, physician, or EMS
5. name of poison, how much was taken, when poisoning occurred
6. save a sample of the vomited material
7. (Any 2 of the following) tickle the back of the victim's throat, give warm salt water, give syrup of ipecac only if recommended by the PCC or a physician
8. to bind the poison so it is not absorbed into the body

9. (Any 4 of the following) unconscious victims, victims who swallow an acid or alkali, victims who swallow petroleum products, victims who are convulsing, victims with burns on lips and mouth
10. remove the victim from the area
11. use large amounts of water to dilute the substance and remove it from the skin
12. (Any 5 of the following) redness and swelling at site, itching, hives, pain, swelling of the throat, difficult or labored breathing, dizziness, change in level of consciousness

CHAPTER 16:6 PROVIDING FIRST AID FOR BURNS

1. an injury caused by fire, heat, chemical agents, radiation, and/or electricity
2. superficial: red, mild swelling, pain

   partial-thickness: blister (or vesicle), skin red or mottled, surface appears wet, swelling, painful

   full-thickness: white or charred appearance, severe pain or painless
3. source of heat, skin area, burn, pain, shock, infection
4. (Any 5 of the following) burns on more than 15 percent of surface of adult (10 percent in child); burns affect face or respiratory tract; victim is having difficulty breathing; burns cover more than one body part; victim has partial-thickness burn and is under 5 or over 60 years of age; burns result from chemicals, explosions, or electricity; all full-thickness burns
5. flush area with large amounts of cool water
6. prevent infection
7. do not break or open them
8. call for medical help immediately and cover with thick sterile dressings
9. flush with large amounts of water for 15–30 minutes or until medical help arrives
10. loss of body fluids (dehydration) occurs quickly

CHAPTER 16:7 PROVIDING FIRST AID FOR HEAT EXPOSURE

1. chemical imbalance that can eventually lead to death
2. muscle pains and spasms resulting from loss of water and salt
3. firm pressure to cramped muscle, small sips of water, victim should rest and move to cool area
4. (Any 6 of the following) pale and clammy skin, diaphoresis, fatigue (or tiredness), weakness, headache, muscle cramps, nausea and/or vomiting, dizziness and/or fainting, normal body temperature or just slightly elevated
5. (Any 3 of the following) moving victim to cooler area; loosening or removing excessive clothing; applying cool, wet cloths; lying victim down with feet elevated 12 inches; giving small sips of water; obtaining medical help as needed
6. approximately normal or just slightly elevated in heat exhaustion and elevated to 105° F or above in heat stroke
7. (Any 3 of the following) high body temperature; red, hot, dry skin; rapid pulse; loss of consciousness
8. convulsions, death
9. (Any 3 of the following) place in tub of cool water; sponge skin with cool water; place ice or cold packs on victim's wrists, ankles, and in axillary and groin area; watch for shock; obtain medical help
10. avoid abnormally warm or hot temperatures for several days, drink sufficient amounts of water and/or electrolyte solutions

CHAPTER 16:8 PROVIDING FIRST AID FOR COLD EXPOSURE

1. wind velocity, amount of humidity, length of exposure
2. (Any 5 of the following) shivering, numbness, weakness, drowsiness, low body temperature, poor coordination, confusion, loss of consciousness
3. (Any 3 of the following) move to warm area, remove wet clothing, warm victim slowly, wrap in blankets or put on dry clothing, give warm liquids
4. freezing of the tissue fluids with damage to the skin and underlying tissues
5. (Any 4 of the following) pale glossy skin, white or grayish-yellow color, blisters, skin cold to touch, numbness, pain that subsides

6. (Any 4 of the following) fingers, toes, ears, nose, cheeks
7. 100°–104° F or 37.8°–40° C
8. rubbing may cause gangrene
9. avoid opening or breaking blisters
10. prevent them from rubbing and causing further injury

CHAPTER 16:9 PROVIDING FIRST AID FOR BONE AND JOINT INJURIES

1. fracture: break in the bone
   dislocation: bone end displaced from a joint or moved out of its normal position
   sprain: injury to tissues surrounding a joint
   strain: overstretching of a muscle
2. closed fracture has no open wound on the skin and an open fracture involves an open wound on the skin
3. (Any 6 of the following) deformities, loss of motion, limited motion, pain and tenderness, swelling, discoloration, bone ends protruding through the skin, hearing bone break or snap, grating sensation, abnormal motion
4. respirations, shock, moving, injury
5. (Any 4 of the following) deformity, limited or abnormal motion, swelling, discoloration, pain and tenderness, shortening or lengthening of affected arm or leg
6. can lead to additional injury to nerves, blood vessels, and other tissues
7. (Any 4 of the following) swelling, pain, discoloration, impaired motion
8. (Any 3 of the following) cold application, elevate affected part, rest, elastic bandage for support
9. cold reduces swelling; warm relaxes the muscles
10. (Any 6 of the following) commercial splints, inflatable, or air, splints, padded boards, cardboard, newspapers, blankets, pillows, boards
11. (Any 3 of the following) long enough to immobilize joint above and below injured area, padded, tied in place, applied so they do not apply pressure to injury
12. make an indentation mark by applying slight pressure with the thumb
13. promote circulation, prevent swelling (or edema), decrease pain
14. (Any 4 of the following) temperature, color, swelling (or edema), amount of pain, color return on nail beds, numbness or tingling
15. immediately loosen the ties holding the splint in place
16. permanent damage resulting in paralysis can occur

CHAPTER 16:10 PROVIDING FIRST AID FOR SPECIFIC INJURIES

1. vision loss, medical help, eye specialist
2. (1) pull upper lid down over lower lid
   (2) raise upper eyelid and use sterile gauze to remove object or gently flush eye with water
3. apply dry sterile dressing and obtain medical help
4. make no attempt to remove it, apply dressings loosely or use a paper cup with a hole in the bottom to support it, keep victim lying flat, obtain medical help
5. wrap it in gauze moistened with cool sterile water or normal saline, put the gauze-wrapped tissue in a plastic bag, and send it to the medical facility with the victim
6. lying on the injured side with head and shoulders elevated slightly to allow fluid to drain
7. (Any 6 of the following) clear or blood-tinged cerebrospinal fluid, loss of consciousness, headache, disturbances in vision, pupils unequal in size, paralysis of muscles, disturbances in speech, convulsions, nausea and/or vomiting
8. (Any 4 of the of the following) keep victim lying flat, treat for shock, watch breathing, allow cerebrospinal fluid to flow, avoid giving any fluids, note length of time victim is unconscious

9. (Any 3 of the following) injuries to nose, change in altitudes, strenuous activity, high blood pressure, rupture of blood vessels after a cold
10. sitting position with head leaning slightly forward
11. airtight, prevent airflow into the wound
12. on injured side with head and chest elevated slightly
13. (Any 4 of the following) pain and tenderness, visibility of protruding organs or open wounds, nausea and/or vomiting, rigidity of abdominal muscles, symptoms of shock
14. flat on the back with a pillow or rolled blanket under the knees to bend the knees slightly, elevate the head and shoulders slightly to aid breathing
15. cover with a large sterile dressing moistened with sterile water or normal saline, make no attempt to replace organs
16. (Any 4 of the following) control severe bleeding, treat for shock, do not remove any penetrating or inserted objects, save any torn tissue, apply cold applications, obtain medical help

CHAPTER 16:11 PROVIDING FIRST AID FOR SUDDEN ILLNESS

1. information from the victim, medical alert bracelets or necklaces, medical information cards
2. (Any 4 of the following) painful pressure under sternum; pain radiating to shoulders, arms, neck, and jaw; intense shortness of breath; pale or cyanotic skin; weak and apprehensive; nausea and/or vomiting; diaphoresis; loss of consciousness
3. (Any 3 of the following) encourage victim to relax, position in comfortable position, obtain medical help, provide treatment for shock, avoid unnecessary stress and movement, reassure victim constantly
4. (Any 6 of the following) numbness, paralysis, pupils of eyes unequal in size, mental confusion, slurred speech, nausea and/or vomiting, difficulty breathing and swallowing, loss of consciousness
5. (Any 3 of the following) maintain respirations, lie victim flat or on side, avoid any fluids by mouth, obtain medical help as quickly as possible, reassure victim, avoid unnecessary stress or movement
6. lying down or sitting in a chair with head at level of knees
7. (Any 3 of the following) lie victim flat, elevate legs and feet if no neck or spine injury is suspected, loosen tight clothing, maintain open airway, bathe face with cool water, check for injuries, get victim up slowly after recovery
8. violent involuntary contraction of muscles
9. self-injury
10. no, can cause injury to your fingers and/or damage victim's teeth or gums
11. force causes the contractions to become more severe
12. diabetic coma, insulin shock
13. (Any 6 of the following) confusion, weakness, dizziness, nausea and/or vomiting, rapid deep respirations, dry and flushed skin, sweet or fruity odor to the breath, loss of consciousness
14. obtain medical assistance as soon as possible
15. (Any 6 of the following) muscle weakness, mental confusion, restlessness or anxiety, diaphoresis, pale and moist skin, hunger pangs, palpitations, coma, convulsions
16. give victim some form of sugar

CHAPTER 16:12 APPLYING DRESSINGS AND BANDAGES

1. sterile covering placed over a wound or an injured part
2. (Any 3 of the following) control bleeding, absorb blood and secretions, prevent infection, ease pain
3. fibers contaminate the wound
4. materials used to hold dressings in place, secure splints, and support and protect body parts
5. bleeding, movement of the dressing, circulation
6. roller gauze, triangular, elastic
7. (Any 3 of the following) sling, bandage for head/scalp, bandage for large body part, secure splints or dressings
8. they can cut off or constrict circulation if applied too tightly or stretched during application

9. (Any 4 of the following) swelling, pale or cyanotic (blue) color, coldness, numbness or tingling, poor return of color to nail beds
10. loosen bandage immediately

CHAPTER 17 PREPARING FOR THE WORLD OF WORK

CHAPTER 17:1 DEVELOPING JOB-KEEPING SKILLS

1. (Any 10 of the following) poor written grammar, poor spelling, poor speech, poor math skills, lack of respect for work, lack of self-initiative, poor personal appearance, not accepting responsibility, excessive tardiness, poor attendance, inability to accept criticism
2. evaluate individual answers: answer should include three job-keeping skills with reasons why student feels competent
3. evaluate individual answers: answer should include three job-keeping skills and two ways to improve competency in each skill

CHAPTER 17:2 WRITING A COVER LETTER AND PREPARING A RÉSUMÉ

1. to obtain an interview
2. computer printed or typewritten, neat, complete, form, spelling, punctuation
3. a. paragraph 1: states purpose for writing and position you are applying for; b. paragraph 2: states why you believe you are qualified; c. paragraph 3: résumé is included; d. paragraph 4: close with a request for an interview, reference as to how employer can contact
4. record of information about an individual
5. a. personal identification: name, address, telephone number, e-mail address
   b. employment objective: title of position you are applying for
   c. educational background: name and address of school, any special training or courses
   d. work or employment experience: name and address of employers, job title, dates employed, and brief description of duties
   e. skills: special knowledge, computer, and work skills
   f. other activities: organizations, offices held, volunteer work, special interests, hobbies, awards
6. no; references should be placed on a separate sheet of paper and given to the employer during the job interview
7. incorrect information can cost you a job
8. standard business envelope that matches the paper or a 9 x 12 envelope to eliminate the need to fold the letter and résumé
9. professional way to highlight your knowledge, abilities, and skills as you prepare for employment or extended education
10. (Any 5 of the following) introductory letter, résumé, skill list and competency level, letter(s) of recommendation, copies of work evaluations, documentation of mastering job-keeping skills, leadership and organization abilities
11. basic skills, thinking skills, personal qualities
12. evaluate individual answers: student should choose three SCANS workplace competencies (manage resources, display interpersonal skills, utilize information, comprehend systems, use technologies) and explain how the competency has been mastered

CHAPTER 17:3 ASSIGNMENT SHEET #1: COMPLETING JOB APPLICATION FORMS

1. to collect specific information
2. (Any 3 of the following) note areas where information is to be placed; read instructions on how to complete form; note whether it should be written, printed or typewritten; check all required information
3. NA or none
4. errors will not impress the potential employer
5. print neatly, black ink, scan, key, accuracy, print

6. a simple half-truth can cost you a job
7. leave it blank, employers judge how well you follow directions
8. obtain his or her permission
9. ensures that you have necessary information with you
10. (Any 3 of the following) completeness of information, spelling, proper answers to questions, errors

CHAPTER 17:4 PARTICIPATING IN A JOB INTERVIEW

1. (Any 2 of the following) allows employer to evaluate you in person, allows employer to obtain additional information, lets employer ascertain whether you meet the job qualifications, tells you about the position in more detail
2. (Any 2 of the following) wallet card, résumé, completed application
3. (Any 4 of the following) conservative dress, clothes fit well, clothes clean and pressed, hair neat, nails clean, teeth clean, effective antiperspirant

   males: coat and tie, clean-shaven

   female: dress, nails—no bright polish, avoid too much makeup
4. 5–10 minutes
5. (Any 8 of the following) greet interviewer by name, remain standing until interviewer asks you to sit, use correct grammar, speak slowly and clearly, be polite, maintain eye contact, answer questions thoroughly, do not smoke or eat candy or chew gum, watch posture and sit straight, smile—avoid giggling, be yourself, be enthusiastic, listen closely, watch awkward habits, do not discuss personal problems or criticize former employers, answer questions truthfully, think before you respond, be proud of yourself, do not immediately ask about salary/fringe benefits/insurance, thank employer
6. send follow-up note, letter, or electronic message (e-mail) to thank employer for interview
7. evaluate students' individual answers

CHAPTER 17:5 DETERMINING NET INCOME

Assign each student a different wage. Then check the answers on this assignment using the following chart. Percentages used are stated. You may have to change figures depending on tax percentages, which vary.

Hourly Wage	40-Hour Week	Federal 15%	State 2%	City 1%	FICA 7.65%	Net Week	Net Month
6.50	260.00	39.00	5.20	2.60	19.89	193.31	773.24
6.75	270.00	40.50	5.40	2.70	20.66	200.74	802.96
7.00	280.00	42.00	5.60	2.80	21.42	208.18	832.72
7.05	282.00	42.30	5.64	2.82	21.57	209.67	838.68
7.10	284.00	42.60	5.68	2.84	21.73	211.15	844.60
7.15	286.00	42.90	5.72	2.86	21.88	212.64	850.56
7.20	288.00	43.20	5.76	2.88	22.03	214.13	856.52
7.25	290.00	43.50	5.80	2.90	22.19	215.61	862.44
7.30	292.00	43.80	5.84	2.92	22.34	217.10	868.40
7.35	294.00	44.10	5.88	2.94	22.49	218.59	874.36
7.40	296.00	44.40	5.92	2.96	22.64	220.08	880.32
7.45	298.00	44.70	5.96	2.98	22.80	221.56	886.24
7.50	300.00	45.00	6.00	3.00	22.95	223.05	892.20
7.55	302.00	45.30	6.04	3.02	23.10	224.54	898.16
7.60	304.00	45.60	6.08	3.04	23.26	226.02	904.08
7.65	306.00	45.90	6.12	3.06	23.41	227.51	910.04
7.70	308.00	46.20	6.16	3.08	23.56	229.00	916.00
7.75	310.00	46.50	6.20	3.10	23.72	230.48	921.92
7.80	312.00	46.80	6.24	3.12	23.87	231.97	927.88
7.85	314.00	47.10	6.28	3.14	24.02	233.46	933.84
7.90	316.00	47.40	6.32	3.16	24.17	234.95	939.80
7.95	318.00	47.70	6.36	3.18	24.33	236.43	945.72
8.00	320.00	48.00	6.40	3.20	24.48	237.92	951.68
8.10	324.00	48.60	6.48	3.24	24.79	240.89	963.56
8.15	326.00	48.90	6.52	3.26	24.94	242.38	969.52
8.20	328.00	49.20	6.56	3.28	25.09	243.87	975.48
8.25	330.00	49.50	6.60	3.30	25.25	245.35	981.40
8.30	332.00	49.80	6.64	3.32	25.40	246.84	987.36
8.35	334.00	50.10	6.68	3.34	25.55	248.33	993.32
8.40	336.00	50.40	6.72	3.36	25.70	249.82	999.28
8.45	338.00	50.70	6.76	3.38	25.86	251.30	1,005.20
8.50	340.00	51.00	6.80	3.40	26.01	252.79	1,011.16
8.60	344.00	51.60	6.88	3.44	26.32	255.76	1,023.04
8.65	346.00	51.90	6.92	3.46	26.47	257.25	1,029.00
8.70	348.00	52.20	6.96	3.48	26.62	258.74	1,034.96
8.75	350.00	52.50	7.00	3.50	26.78	260.22	1,040.88
8.80	352.00	52.80	7.04	3.52	26.93	261.71	1,046.84
8.85	354.00	53.10	7.08	3.54	27.08	263.20	1,052.80
8.90	356.00	53.40	7.12	3.56	27.23	264.69	1,058.76
8.95	358.00	53.70	7.16	3.58	27.39	266.17	1,064.68
9.00	360.00	54.00	7.20	3.60	27.54	267.66	1,070.64
9.25	370.00	55.50	7.40	3.70	28.31	275.09	1,100.36
9.50	380.00	57.00	7.60	3.80	29.07	282.53	1,130.12
9.75	390.00	58.50	7.80	3.90	29.84	289.96	1,159.84
10.00	400.00	60.00	8.00	4.00	30.60	297.40	1,189.60
10.25	410.00	61.50	8.20	4.10	31.37	304.83	1,219.32
10.50	420.00	63.00	8.40	4.20	32.13	312.27	1,249.08
10.75	430.00	64.50	8.60	4.30	32.90	319.70	1,278.80
11.00	440.00	66.00	8.80	4.40	33.66	327.14	1,308.56
11.25	450.00	67.50	9.00	4.50	34.43	334.57	1,338.28
11.50	460.00	69.00	9.20	4.60	35.19	342.01	1,368.04
11.75	470.00	70.50	9.40	4.70	35.96	349.44	1,397.76
12.00	480.00	72.00	9.60	4.80	36.72	356.88	1,427.52
12.25	490.00	73.50	9.80	4.90	37.49	364.31	1,457.24
12.50	500.00	75.00	10.00	5.00	38.25	371.75	1,487.00

CHAPTER 17: 6 CALCULATING A BUDGET

Grade this assignment on an individual basis. Make sure students use realistic amounts in each category. Check total amounts. Make sure expenses equal net monthly income.

CHAPTER 18 DENTAL ASSISTANT SKILLS

CHAPTER 18:1 IDENTIFYING THE STRUCTURES AND TISSUES OF A TOOTH

1. A. crown
   B. cervix or cemento-enamel junction
   C. root
   D. apex with apical foramen
   E. enamel
   F. dentin
   G. pulp in pulp chamber
   H. free gingiva
   I. alveolar process
   J. attached gingiva
   K. cementum
   L. pulp canal
   M. periodontal ligament
2. 20
3. 6 months of age
4. (Any 2 of the following) maintain proper spacing, mastication, speech
5. 5 to 6 years of age
6. 32
7. mixed
8. a. dentin
   b. apical foramen
   c. pulp
   d. cervix or cemento-enamel junction
   e. crown
   f. enamel
   g. cementum
   h. root
   i. pulp
   j. enamel
9. periodontium
10. (1) D (2) A (3) D (4) C (5) A (6) D (7) B (8) D (9) B and C (10) D

CHAPTER 18:2 IDENTIFYING THE TEETH

1. Primary or Deciduous Teeth: see Figure 18-3 in information section of textbook on Identifying the Teeth
2. Permanent or Succedaneous Teeth: see Figure 18-4 in information section of textbook on Identifying the Teeth
3. (1) B (2) A (3) C (4) D (5) B (6) A, D (7) C (8) B (9) B (10) D (11) C (12) A
4. transverse, or horizontal, plane
5. midsagittal, median, midline

CHAPTER 18:3 IDENTIFYING TEETH USING THE UNIVERSAL/NATIONAL NUMBERING SYSTEM AND FEDERATION DENTAIRE INTERNATIONAL (FDI) SYSTEM

1. Primary teeth labeled by Universal/National Numbering System: teeth labeled from A–T, see figure 18-5 in textbook
2. A max. rt. 2nd molar H
   G max. lft. lateral incisor S
   K mand. lft. 2nd molar N
   P mand. rt. central incisor B
   T mand. rt. 2nd molar R
   I max. lft. 1st molar O
   C max. rt. cuspid D
   E max. rt. central incisor L
   M mand. lft. cuspid F
   Q mand. rt. lateral incisor J

3. d-3 max. rt. cuspid
   d-10 mand.rt. 1st molar
   d-8 max. lft. cuspid
   d-14 mand. lft. lateral incisor
   d-6 max. lft. central incisor
   d-11 mand. lft. 2nd molar

4. Permanent teeth labeled by Universal/National Numbering System: teeth labeled from 1–32 see Figure 18-6 in book

5.

1 max. rt. 3rd molar	7	23 mand. lft. lateral incisor	26
8 max. rt. central incisor	29	17 mand. lft.. 3rd molar	21
15 max. lft.. 2nd molar	19	12 max. lft. 1st bicuspid	9
20 mand. lft. 2nd bicuspid	24	30 mand. rt.1st molar	31
28 mand. rt. 1st bicuspid	11	3 max. rt. 1st molar	22
32 mand. rt. 3rd molar	6	25 mand. rt. central incisor	2
16 max. lft. 3rd molar	18	10 max. lft. lateral incisor	27
4 max. rt. 2nd bicuspid	13	5 max. rt. 1st bicuspid	14

6. Primary teeth labeled according to Federation Dentaire International (FDI) System, see Figure 18-7 in textbook

7.

51 max. rt. central incisor	55	53 max. rt. cuspid	61
74 mand. lft. 1st molar	73	72 mand. lft. lateral incisor	75
63 max. lft. cuspid	81	65 max. lft. 2nd molar	52
85 mand. rt. 2nd molar	62	54 max. rt. 1st molar	83
82 mand. rt. lateral incisor	84	71 mand. lft. central incisor	64

8. Permanent teeth labeled according to Federation Dentaire International (FDI) System, see figure 18-8 in textbook

9.

11 max. rt. central incisor	12	18 max. rt. 3rd molar	44
23 max. lft. cuspid	45	41 mand. rt. central incisor	31
28 max. lft. 3rd molar	37	24 max. lft. 1st bicuspid	16
47 mand. rt. 2nd molar	21	36 mand. lft. 1st molar	25
35 mand. lft. 2nd bicuspid	46	14 max. rt. 1st bicuspid	34
22 max. lft. lateral incisor	32	33 mand. lft. cuspid	48
15 max. rt. 2nd bicuspid	13	42 mand. rt. lateral incisor	17
43 mand. rt. cuspid	26	38 mand. lft. 3rd molar	27

CHAPTER 18:4 IDENTIFYING THE SURFACES OF THE TEETH

A.

1. incisal	I	7. mesioincisal	MI
2. distal	D	8. distoincisal	DI
3. lingual	Li	9. linguoincisal	LiI
4. medial	M	10. distolingual	DLi
5. labial	La	11. mesiolinguoincisal	MLiI
6. mesiolingual	MLi	12. distolinguoincisal	DLiI

B.

1. buccal	B	10. distolingual	DLi
2. occlusal	O	11. linguoocclusal	LiO
3. mesial	M	12. mesiolingual	MLi
4. distal	D	13. mesioocclusal	MO
5. lingual	Li	14. mesiobuccoocclusal	MBO
6. mesiobuccal	MB	15. distobuccoocclusal	DBO
7. buccoocclusal	BO	16. distolinguoocclusal	DLiO
8. distobuccal	DB	17. mesiolinguoocclusal	MLiO
9. distoocclusal	DO		

CHAPTER 18:5 ASSIGNMENT SHEET #1 CHARTING CONDITIONS OF THE TEETH

Following charted on dental card:

1/20/—		Ex, FMXR, Pro, and FI
1/23/—	2	AM to O
	8	Comp to MLaI, Dycal
3/10/—		BWXR–4
	11	RCT
5/3/—	12	AM to MOD
5/20/—	17	Ext
6/2/—	23	Comp to DLinI
7/12/—		Ex, Pro, Al. Imp. Mandibular
7/30/—	4	Am to B
8/15/—	30	Cr-Gold

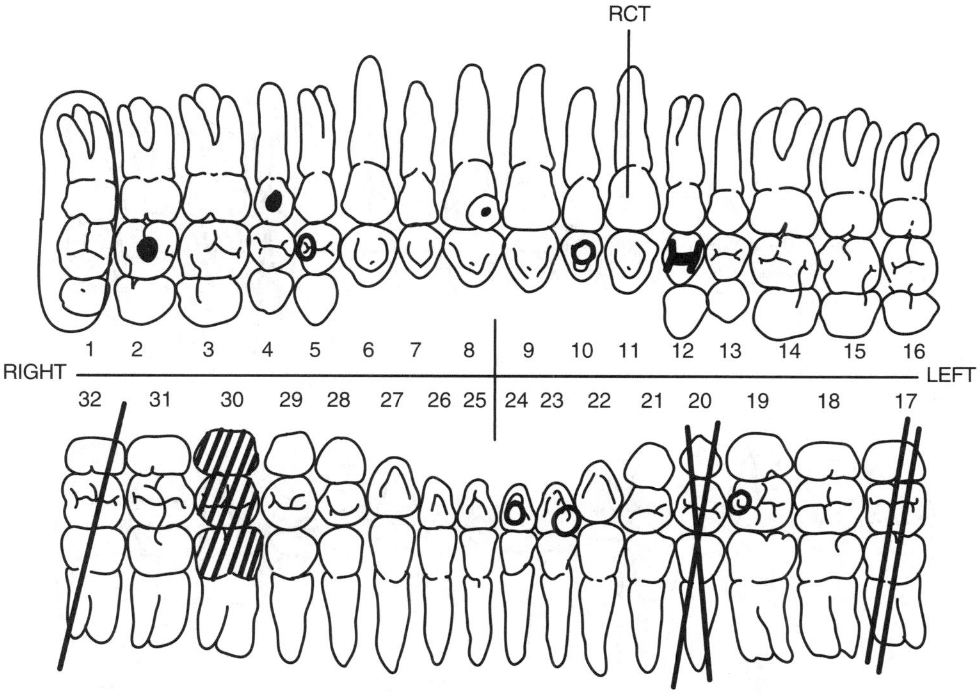

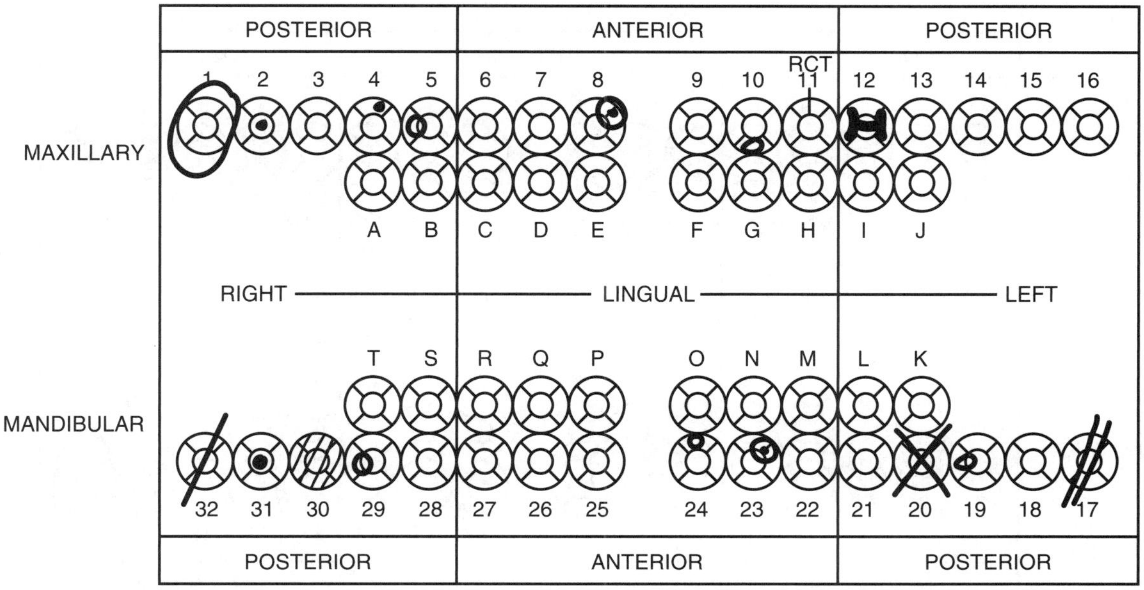

CHAPTER 18:5 ASSIGNMENT SHEET #2 CHARTING CONDITIONS OF THE TEETH

Following charted on dental card:

1/1/—		Ex, FMXR
1/23/—	20	AM to MO
1/30/—	3	AM to MOD
2/3/—	11	RCT
6/2/—		Ex, BWXR, Pro
7/4/—	8	Comp to MLinI, Dycal
8/9/—	6	RB Imp.
8/20/—	6	Cr-Porcelain
2/11/—		Ex, Pro, BWXR–4
3/8/—	22	AM to Lin
4/6/—	31	AM to MO
4/28/—	24	Comp to Lin

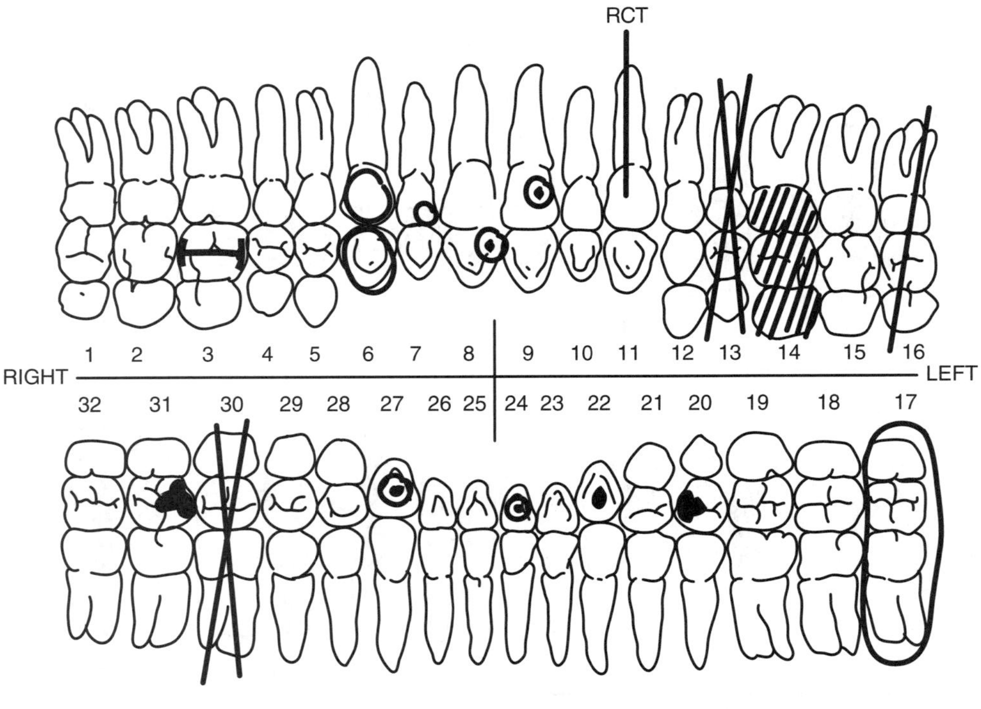

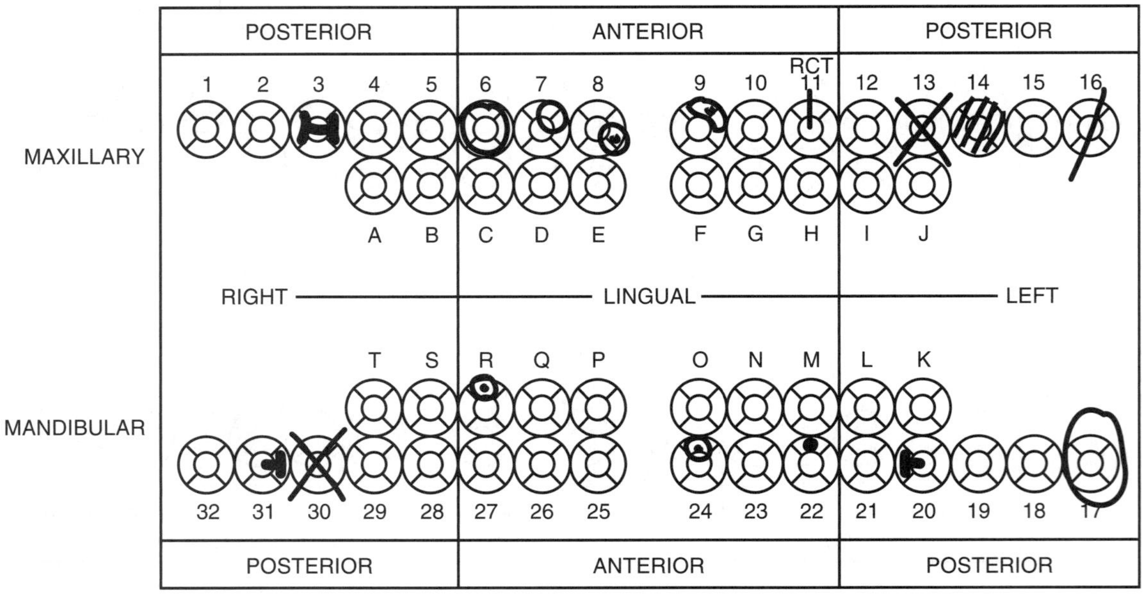

CHAPTER 18:5 ASSIGNMENT SHEET #3 CHARTING CONDITIONS OF THE TEETH

Following charted on dental card:

5/7/—		FMXR, PRO, Ex
6/1/—	20	AM to DO, I.R.M.
6/15/—	17	Ext.
7/2/—	6	R.B. Imp.
7/20/—	6	Cr. Porc.
10/1/—		Ex, PRO, BWXR–4
10/15/—	11	Comp to LaI
10/22/—	13	AM to DO
11/3/—	4	AM to DB
3/3/—		EX, FMXR, PRO
3/20/—	22	Comp to Lin, Dycal
4/2/—	29	AM to MO, IRM
4/15/—	25	RCT
5/3/—	30	AM on O

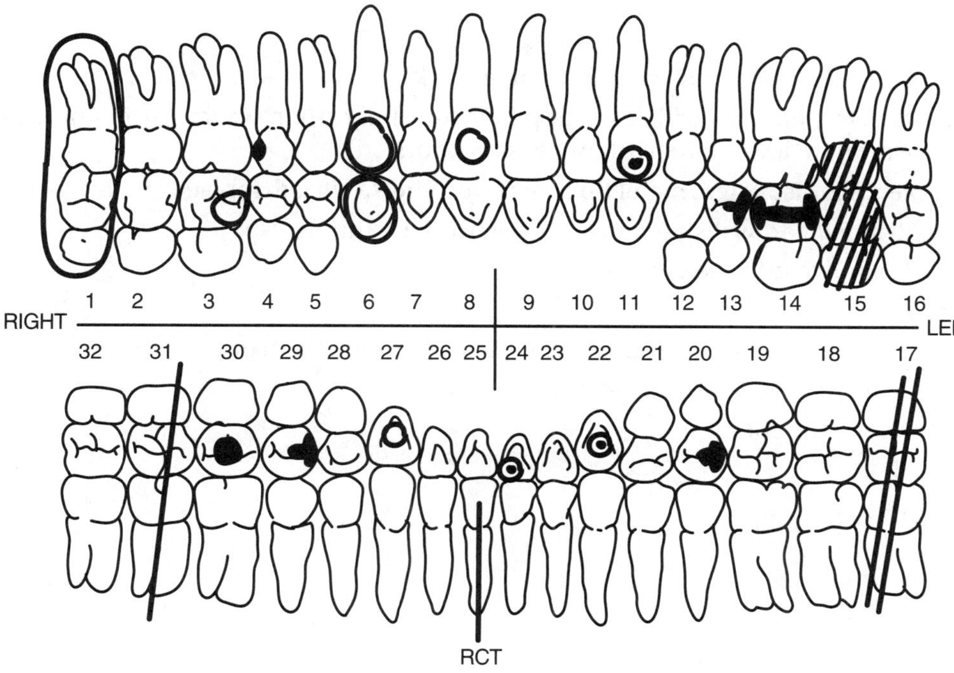

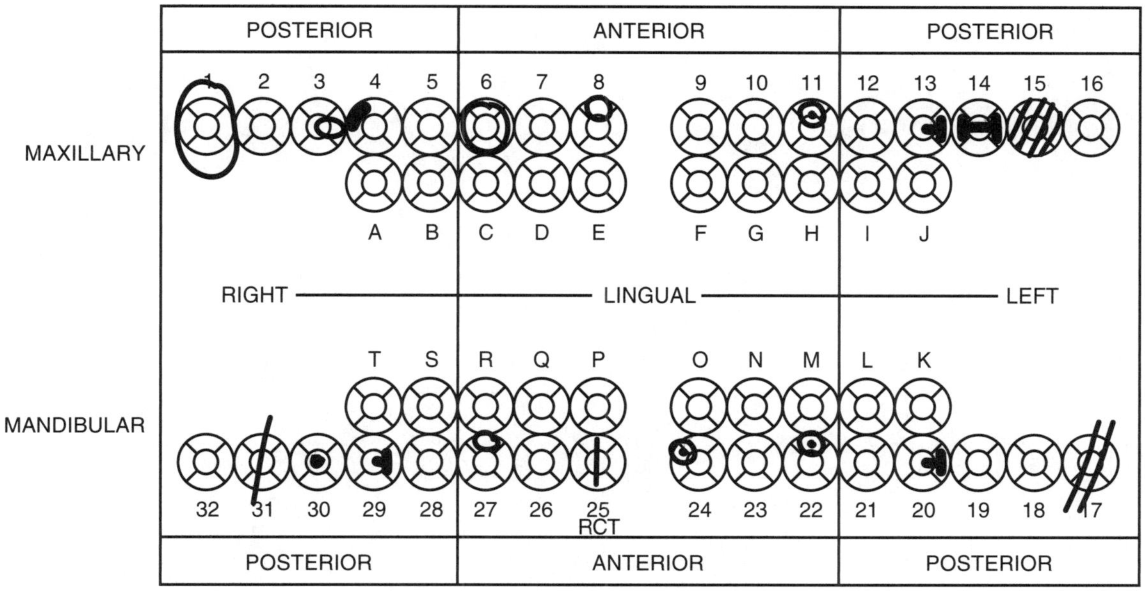

CHAPTER 18:6 OPERATING AND MAINTAINING DENTAL EQUIPMENT

1. blood, saliva, body fluids, standard precautions, protective, disinfect, sterilize, gloves, disinfected
2. a. dental light: illuminate oral cavity
   b. dental chair: position the patient
   c. air compressor: provides air pressure to run handpieces
   d. oral evacuation system: remove particles and liquid from oral cavity
   e. air-water syringe: provides air, water, or a combination
   f. saliva ejector: provides low-volume suction to remove saliva and other fluids from the mouth
   g. high-velocity evacuator: remove particles, debris, and large amounts of liquid from oral cavity
   h. cuspidor: allows patient to expectorate particles and water
   i. low-speed handpiece: carries removal and fine finishing work
   j. high-speed handpiece: cutting and preparation of the tooth during dental procedures
3. 30–50 inches; prevents formation of scratches on light shield
4. doctor and assistant can position themselves close to patient; prevent movement while patient is getting in or out of the chair
5. 100, 120
6. check oil level in oil reservoir, drain water from main tank
7. catches large particles; empty particles into paper towel and then wash, rinse, and dry trap; prevent growth of organisms and development of unpleasant odors
8. plastic disposable tip is discarded, metal tip is removed and sterilized, replaced with a sterile tip
9. remove barrier, disinfect, draw disinfecting solution through tubing
10. trap large particles drawn into the evacuator
11. prevent sticking
12. contra-angle: cutting and polishing; prophylaxis angle: clean the teeth or polishing restorations
13. scrubbed thoroughly, rinsed, dried, and sterilized
14. read manufacturer's instructions

CHAPTER 18:7 IDENTIFYING DENTAL INSTRUMENTS AND PREPARING DENTAL TRAYS

1. set up for particular patient or preset by procedure
2. proper sequence, order of use
3. a. prophylactic or oral examination: basic examination and cleaning of the teeth
   b. amalgam restoration: amalgam restorative procedure
   c. composite restoration: placement of composite or anterior restorative
   d. surgical extraction: removing or extracting teeth
4. a. blade, b. nib, c. point, d. shank, e. shaft
5. Answers to crossword puzzle

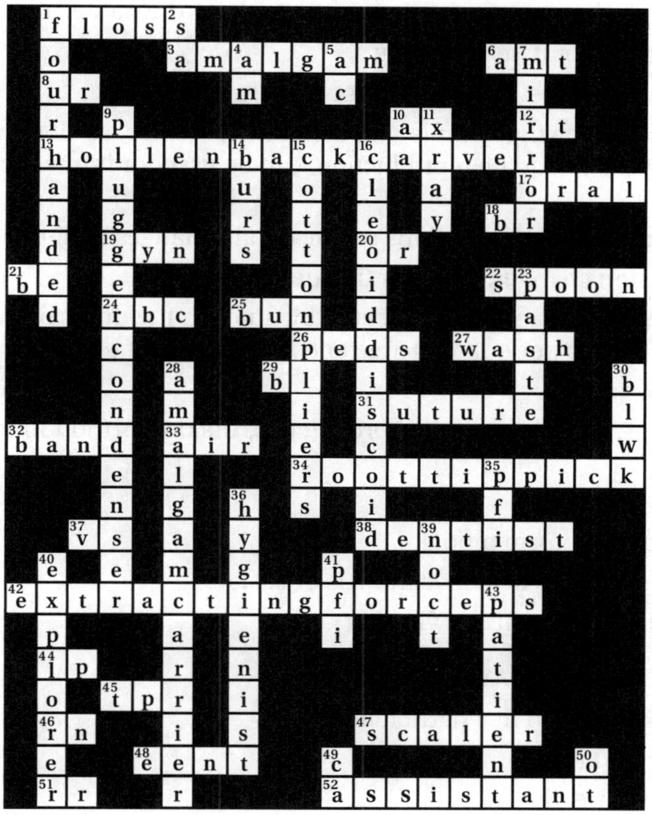

CHAPTER 18:8 POSITIONING A PATIENT IN THE DENTAL CHAIR

1. supine, lying down
2. allows the dentist and assistant closer access to the oral cavity
3. to a height that will allow the doctor to be seated comfortably by the chair with the patient's head above the doctor's lap
4. when patient gets in chair, when patient gets out of chair
5. allow the patient time to adjust to the change in position; avoid dizziness, discomfort, and fear
6. unexpected movements can frighten the patient
7. protect the patient's clothing
8. plastic side, plastic prevents moisture from soaking through to patient's clothing
9. protects the patient's eyes from sprays and fluids that may be present during a dental procedure
10. 30–50 inches, illuminates the mouth, shine in the patient's eyes

CHAPTER 18:9 DEMONSTRATING BRUSHING AND FLOSSING TECHNIQUES

1. prevent decay or carious lesions, remove plaque, prevent halitosis or bad breath
2. all patients, slowly, clearly, repeat, stress
3. 45° angle, vibrating

4. chewing or biting, facial, lingual, one side, other side
5. side surfaces (interproximal surfaces)
6. soft bristled; will not injure gum or gingival tissue
7. when bristles are frayed or worn
8. clean teeth and provide pleasant taste
9. aids in preventing decay
10. waxed and unwaxed; whichever type doctor prefers

CHAPTER 18:10 TAKING IMPRESSIONS AND POURING MODELS

1. impression: negative reproduction of a tooth, several teeth, or the dental arch
2. to form model of area for restorative treatment
3. alginate, rubber base, or silicones (polysiloxane or polyvinylsiloxane)
4. advantages: (any 3 of the following) simple and economical to use, setting time controlled by water temperature, adequate strength, adequate reproduction, can be used for impressions of the teeth and/or tissue, easily cleaned

   disadvantages: not good for final impressions or fine detail, changes in dimension, tears or breaks easily
5. not as subject to dimension changes, good for fine detail
6. (Any 3 of the following) easy cleanup, not affected by fluids in the oral cavity, highly accurate impression, retains shape and size for long period, odor-free and has a pleasant taste
7. positive reproduction of arches or teeth
8. construction of dentures, partials, or other prosthetics; making orthodontic appliances, mouth guards, and custom trays
9. plaster, stone
10. stronger, more regular and uniform model
11. moisture contamination leads to defective models or casts
12. stir and spatulate carefully, place mix on vibrator

CHAPTER 18:11 MAKING CUSTOM TRAYS

1. impression trays that are made to fit a particular patient
2. preliminary impression and model
3. base, custom tray, fitted perfectly
4. curing; causes material to become pliable so it can be fitted to the contour of the preliminary model
5. light-cured resins do not set, or become hard, until they are exposed to a light in a special curing oven
6. plastic- or wax-lined disposable paper cup and tongue blades
7. coat with petroleum jelly
8. they can be vacuum-formed to make a custom tray

CHAPTER 18:12 MAINTAINING AND LOADING AN ANESTHETIC ASPIRATING SYRINGE

1. sensation of feeling pain has been decreased or eliminated
2. decrease pain or discomfort caused by injection; to mucous membranes as spray, liquid, gel, or ointment
3. block: near main nerve trunk, mandibular

   infiltration/field: terminal nerve branches of teeth, maxillary or anterior mandibular
4. Lidocaine or Xylocaine
5. (Any 2 of the following) decrease size of blood vessels, prolong effect, reduce bleeding; epinephrine
6. a. glass: no cracks or chips; b. solution: clear in color; c. rubber plunger: basically level with or just slightly below top; d. bubbles: small bubbles only; e. aluminum cap: clean, no rust
7. use sterile pad with 70 percent ethyl alcohol or 91 percent isopropyl; disinfectant passes through rubber diaphragm and contaminates solution
8. be sure needle has not penetrated a blood vessel

9. (1) thumb ring, (2) finger grip, (3) spring, (4) guide bearing, (5) piston with harpoon, (6) barrel, (7) needle adaptor
10. wash, rinse, sterilize in autoclave
11. take apart, check parts, replace worn or defective parts, lubricate threaded joints
12. leakproof, puncture-resistant sharps box; bent; broken; recapped

CHAPTER 18:13 MIXING DENTAL CEMENTS AND BASES

1. a. liner: material used to cover, seal, or line exposed tooth tissue; example: varnish
   b. base: protective material placed over pulpal area of tooth to reduce irritation and thermal shock; example: calcium hydroxide, zinc oxide eugenol, zinc phosphate, carboxylate
   c. cement: material used to seal inlays, orthodontic appliances, crowns, bridges in place; example: zinc phosphate, carboxylates
   d. temporary: material used as a restorative for a short time; example: zinc oxide eugenol
2. (3 examples for each) a. varnish: Copal, Copalite, Varnal, or Handi-Liner; b. zinc oxide eugenol: IRM, Cavitec, Wonder Pak, or Interval; c. calcium hydroxide: Dycal, Preline, Hypocal, or Dropsin; d. carboxylates: Durelon, Hybond, or Tylock-Plus
3. no; interferes with setting reaction of the materials
4. no; it is water soluble
5. thermally protective base, cement for gold restorations
6. improper techniques can lead to a poor base or cement and shorten life of restoration
7. read manufacturer's directions
8. contamination of a container can destroy the entire contents

CHAPTER 18:14 PREPARING RESTORATIVE MATERIALS—AMALGAM AND COMPOSITE

1. process of replacing a diseased portion of a tooth or lost tooth by artificial means
2. composite, amalgam
3. silver: high strength, low flow, high expansion, rapid setting, silver color

   tin: counterbalances silver, reduces expansion, slows setting time, reduces strength, increases ability of alloy to combine with mercury, allows restoration to be carved

   copper: increases strength, hardness, low flow, increases expansion, stabilizes other metals

   zinc: removes oxides and other impurities
4. mercury
5. (Any 3 of the following) wear personal protective equipment (PPE); store in well-sealed, unbreakable container; clean up spills immediately; discard mercury-contaminated items in a sealed polyethylene bag
6. submerged in a tightly sealed, unbreakable jar containing sulfur water, glycerin, or mineral oil
7. mixing process used to combine mercury with amalgam alloy
8. improved appearance, increased strength, ability to withstand chemical actions caused by mouth fluids
9. when material is exposed to curing light
10. etching roughens surface so composite will adhere and bond more securely to tooth tissue, bonding agent helps composite adhere to tooth

CHAPTER 18:15 DEVELOPING AND MOUNTING DENTAL RADIOGRAPHS (X-RAYS)

1. radiolucent; pulp; caries; radiopaque; enamel; dentin; metallic restorations
2. a. bite-wings, b. periapical, c. panoramic
3. stops the X-ray beams once they have passed through the teeth structures
4. exposure to light will destroy film
5. keeps the silver from settling and keeps it suspended on the surface of the film
6. 68° F, or 20° C
7. break down exposed silver; alkaline

8. stop developing process; acid
9. facial (buccal or labial)
10. lingual (tongue)

CHAPTER 19 LABORATORY ASSISTANT SKILLS

CHAPTER 19:1 OPERATING THE MICROSCOPE

1. eyepiece(s)
2. body tube
3. arm
4. coarse adjustment
5. fine adjustment
6. base
7. illuminating light
8. condenser and iris diaphragm
9. stage with side clips
10. objectives
11. revolving nosepiece
12. electron beams
13. to detect antibodies and specific organisms
14. crack slide and/or damage objective
15. adjust iris diaphragm
16. other materials scratch delicate glass
17. brings the slide into rough focus
18. get precise and clear image
19. concentrates light so object can be seen
20. a. 40, b. 100, c. 400
21. a. 80, b. 200, c. 800
22. covered with a dust cover or stored in a dust-free closet

CHAPTER 19:2 OBTAINING AND HANDLING CULTURES

1. to identify the causative agent of a disease
2. prevent contamination from other sources
3. special solid medium that provides both nourishment and moisture for the organism
4. a. resistant: antibiotic would not work against the organism
   b. sensitive: antibiotic would work against the organism
5. doctor can determine which antibiotic or medication to give the patient for the disease or infection
6. slide is held over a source of heat for a very brief period of time; heat causes organisms to stick to the slide
7. gentian violet or crystal violet: primary stain, stains gram-positive organisms; one minute
   iodine: sets the primary dye or makes it adhere to the organisms on the slide; one minute
   ethyl alcohol or acetone-alcohol: removes gentian violet from gram-negative organisms; until solution running off the slide is no longer purple in color
   safranin: counterstain, stains gram-negative organisms; 30–60 seconds
8. provides another method for identifying organisms
9. identify organisms quickly so effective antibiotics can be started immediately
10. gloves, lab coat or apron, mask, protective eyewear

CHAPTER 19:3 PUNCTURING THE SKIN TO OBTAIN CAPILLARY BLOOD

1. skin puncture, venipuncture, arterial puncture
2. in some states, health occupations students are not permitted to perform procedures that involve obtaining blood
3. clean skin with alcohol, use sterile lancet, cover puncture with sterile gauze
4. (Any 5 of the following) do not use thumb, index finger, or pinkie finger; check edema; check callouses; check scars; check rashes; check sores; make sure skin is warm and pink; do not use if cyanotic
5. 2–4 mm
6. across, right angles
7. contaminated with alcohol, perspiration, excess tissue fluid, and other substances
8. until the blood flow ceases
9. diseases can be transmitted by improper handling of blood samples
10. place in a leakproof, puncture-resistant sharps box

CHAPTER 19:4 PERFORMING A MICROHEMATOCRIT

1. a blood test that measures the volume of packed red blood cells in the blood
2. oxygen, carbon dioxide, 4.5 to 5.5 million per cubic millimeter of blood
3. requires less blood, done in a shorter period of time than other methods for determining hematocrit
4. red blood cells, buffy coat (white blood cells and platelets), plasma
5. fighting infections; 5,000 to 9,000 per cubic millimeters of blood; 8,000
6. prevents the blood from clotting
7. prevents the blood from running out of the tube during centrifuging
8. 46.5 percent
9. a. 35–45 percent; b. 40–55 percent; c. 51–61 percent; d. 34–42 percent
10. anemia, severe bleeding
11. polycythemia, dehydration, burns
12. test is used to diagnose disease, false results can lead to improper diagnosis and care
13. repeat the test
14. the physician

CHAPTER 19:5 MEASURING HEMOGLOBIN

1. substance found in red blood cells
2. carries oxygen and carbon dioxide
3. the oxygen-carrying capacity of blood or grams of hemoglobin per 100 mL of blood
4. special instrument that measures the hemoglobin content in blood
5. destroying red blood cells; hemoglobin is released into the solution surrounding the cells
6. blood changes in appearance from cloudy to clear (or transparent)
7. a. 13–18 grams, b. 12–16 grams, c. 16–23 grams, d. 10–14 grams
8. anemia; polycythemia
9. repeat the test
10. it does not depend on an individual's ability to compare color intensities

CHAPTER 19:6 PREPARING AND STAINING A BLOOD FILM OR SMEAR

1. a spreader is used to spread a small drop of blood into a thin layer on a slide
2. 100, total, type, percentage
3. it is an aid in making a diagnosis because certain types of white blood cells increase after specific infections
4. form, structure, relative number, erythrocytes, leukocytes, platelets, shapes
5. certain types of leukemia

6. contaminants will interfere with and even distort the appearance of the cells
7. alcohol
8. stains cells, fixes smear
9. fixative, one second, staining, one second, four to five, manufacturer's
10. faster, requires less than one minute to complete

CHAPTER 19:7 TESTING FOR BLOOD TYPES

1. antigens
2. a. type A, b. type AB, c. type O, d. type B, e. type Rh positive, f. type Rh negative
3. a. hemolyze: red blood cells dissolve and go into solution, releasing hemoglobin
   b. agglutinate: red blood cells clump together
4. typing and crossmatch
5. typing determines the ABO and Rh factors and crossmatch checks for other incompatibilities
6. test to check for antibodies, done to avoid incompatible reaction
7. when woman is Rh negative and fetus is Rh positive
8. a. type AB positive, b. type O positive, c. type A negative, d. type B positive

CHAPTER 19:8 PERFORMING AN ERYTHROCYTE SEDIMENTATION RATE

1. distance that red blood cells fall or settle in a specific period of time
2. an anticoagulant (oxalate or sequestrene), to prevent clotting of blood
3. holds the tube in an exact vertical position
4. 20 minute, one hour
5. Westergren system: completely closed system that eliminates the manual transfer of blood that can result in leakage, overfilling, and spraying from the transfer pipette
6. a. 0 to 20 mm/hr
   b. 0 to 9 mm/hr
   c. 0 to 20 mm/hr for adult females younger than 50 years and 0 to 30 mm/hr for females older than 50
   d. 0 to 15 mm/hr for adult males younger than 50 years and 0 to 20 mm/hr for males older than 50
7. (Any 5 of the following) infections, carcinoma (or cancer), leukemia, rheumatic fever, rheumatoid arthritis, viral hepatitis, pregnant or menstruating female
8. (Any 4 of the following) polycythemia, certain types of heart disease, congestive heart failure, severe liver disease, sickle cell anemia

CHAPTER 19:9 MEASURING BLOOD-SUGAR (GLUCOSE) LEVEL

1. glucose, insulin, bloodstream, kidneys, urine
2. a. hyperglycemia: high blood sugar
   b. glycosuria: excess amounts of sugar in the urine
   c. hypoglycemia: low blood sugar
3. patient has nothing to eat or drink for 8 to 12 hours, venipuncture is done, serum level of glucose is checked
4. 70 to 110 mg/deciliter of blood is checked
5. how well a person metabolizes a calculated amount of glucose
6. fasting blood sugar measures the current level of glucose in the blood, glycohemoglobin test measures the average blood sugar level for the previous two to three months
7. (Any 4 of the following) increased accuracy, can be done at any time, detects both low and high glucose levels, better regulation of insulin dosage, improved control of diabetes
8. strips of plastic with chemical reagent pads
9. color change
10. compare color to color chart on bottle, place in glucose meter for reading

11. strips are very sensitive to heat, light, and moisture
12. dark, dry, and cool area but not refrigerated
13. chemicals and moisture on the skin can cause inaccurate results; chemicals can burn or injure the skin
14. time and procedure methods vary with different strips
15. lens paper or water can be used to clean screen, disinfectant can be put on areas unless prohibited by manufacturer

CHAPTER 19:10 TESTING URINE

1. 1000–2000, polyuria, oliguria, anuria
2. straw yellow to amber; pale: dilute; clear red: hemoglobin or RBC destruction; cloudy red: RBCs present (hematuria); yellow or beer-brown: bilirubin or bile pigment
3. clear; (any 3 of the following) pus, mucus, white blood cells, old specimen
4. faintly aromatic; ammonia: old specimen; fruity: acetone or ketones or diabetes; foul: bacteria or infection
5. 5.5–8.0, mildly acid
6. 1.005 to 1.030; increased: (any 3 of the following) diabetes mellitus, concentrated urine, low fluid intake, dehydration; decreased: (any 3 of the following) renal disease, diluted urine, high fluid intake, diuretic medications
7. (Any 8 of the following) glucose: diabetes; albumin: kidney disease; acetones-ketones: starvation, diabetes, mellitus, or high-fat diet; blood: kidney disease or infection; pus: infection; bacteria: infection; RBCs: kidney disease or bleeding in urinary tract; WBCs: infection if large amount; bilirubin: liver disease, bile duct obstruction, or hepatitis; urobilinogen: liver disease or destruction of red blood cells (hemolytic diseases)
8. physical, chemical, microscopic
9. color, odor, transparency, specific gravity
10. (Any 6 of the following) pH, protein, glucose, ketone, bilirubin, urobilinogen, blood
11. to spin out solid particles and form urinary sediment
12. within one hour after it is collected

CHAPTER 19:11 USING REAGENT STRIPS TO TEST URINE

1. by the kidney as part of urine
2. firm plastic strips with small pads containing chemical reactants
3. chemicals react with reactant on strip and produce a color change
4. store in dry, cool, dark area; keep moisture-absorbent pad in the bottle; close bottle immediately after use
5. contact with skin can lead to an inaccurate test, chemicals can burn or injure the skin
6. chemical reactants are effective only for a certain period of time; no; inaccurate test results will occur
7. (Any 3 of the following) diet, medications, kidney disease, starvation, diabetes mellitus
8. a. protein: kidney disease
   b. glucose: diabetes mellitus
   c. ketones (acetones): diabetes, starvation, fasting, dieting, high-fat diet, metabolic disorders
   d. blood: injury, infection, or disease in kidneys and/or urinary tract
   e. bilirubin: liver disease such as hepatitis or bile duct obstruction
   f. urobilinogen: heart, spleen, liver or hemolytic disease
   g. phenalanine: phenylketonuria (PKU)
9. (Any 3 strips for each substance)
   a. pH: Bili-Labstix, Combistix, Labstix, Multistix
   b. glucose: Bili-Labstix, Chemstrip-GK, Chemstrip-GP, Clinistix, Combistix, Diastix, Keto-Diastix, Labstix, Multistix, Uristix
   c. protein: Albustix, Bili-Labstix, Chemstrip-GP, Combistix, Labstix, Multistix, Uristix
   d. ketones: Bili-Labstix, Chemstrip-GK, Keto-Diastix, Ketostix, Labstix, Multistix
   e. blood: Bili-Labstix, Hemastix, Labstix, Multistix
10. lists substances to be tested, gives correct time interval for reading each reaction
11. to make sure strips produce accurate results; urine control solution with predetermined results is tested, and measurements must match predetermined range

12. it is more accurate than the human eye
13. fresh urine specimen
14. within one hour after collection; results are more accurate

CHAPTER 19:12 MEASURING SPECIFIC GRAVITY

1. weight of urine compared with the weight of an equal amount of distilled water
2. 1.005 to 1.030 with most specimens ranging between 1.010 and 1.025
3. (Any 3 of the following) excessive fluid intake, kidney disease in which kidneys cannot concentrate urine, diuretic medications, diabetes insipidus
4. (Any 3 of the following) low fluid intake, dehydration, excessive fluid loss, kidney disease, diabetes mellitus
5. a. 1.001
   b. 1.005
   c. 1.008
   d. 1.012
   e. 1.015
   f. 1.019
   g. 1.024
   h. 1.029
   i. 1.034
   j. 1.038
6. one drop, ocular, eyepiece, accuracy, strips, solutions

CHAPTER 19:13 PREPARING URINE FOR MICROSCOPIC EXAMINATION

1. examine the solid materials (urinary sediment) suspended in the urine
2. fresh, first-voided morning specimen is more concentrated and more likely to contain abnormal substances
3. certain substances disintegrate rapidly in warm specimens
4. kept cold
5. spins urine, causing solid material to settle to the bottom
6. sediment
7. cover slip will float; empty space under cover slip
8. drying occurs quickly, which can result in distortions in the shape and size of substances present
9. per low power field, per high power field
10. CLIA-waived, moderately complex, legally qualified

CHAPTER 20 MEDICAL ASSISTANT SKILLS

CHAPTER 20:1 MEASURING/RECORDING HEIGHT AND WEIGHT

1. to determine if a patient is overweight or underweight
2. allows a physician to check the child's growth and compare it to the average percentiles of other children the same age
3. hydrocephalus, microencephaly
4. to determine the progression of chronic obstructive pulmonary diseases (COPDs) such as emphysema
5. (Any 4 of the following) use the same scale each day, make sure the scale is balanced, weigh the patient at the same time each day, weigh the patient early in the morning before any food or liquids have been consumed, make sure the patient is wearing the same amount of clothing each day, ask the patient to void, or empty the bladder
6. answer will be individualized; student should tell the patient that the physician will determine whether weight is excessive

7. A. 2	E. $6\frac{3}{4}$	I. $12\frac{1}{4}$	M. 18	
B. $3\frac{1}{4}$	F. $8\frac{1}{2}$	J. $13\frac{3}{4}$	N. $19\frac{1}{4}$	
C. $4\frac{1}{4}$	G. $10\frac{1}{4}$	K. $15\frac{1}{2}$	O. $20\frac{1}{2}$	
D. 6	H. 11	L. $16\frac{3}{4}$		
8. A. 52	D. 56	G. $210\frac{1}{4}$	J. $213\frac{3}{4}$	M. 268
B. $53\frac{1}{4}$	E. $56\frac{3}{4}$	H. 211	K. $265\frac{1}{2}$	N. $269\frac{1}{4}$
C. $54\frac{1}{4}$	F. $208\frac{1}{2}$	I. $212\frac{1}{4}$	L. $266\frac{3}{4}$	O. $270\frac{1}{2}$
9. A. $47\frac{1}{2}$	D. $44\frac{1}{4}$	G. $40\frac{1}{2}$	J. $37\frac{1}{4}$	M. $54\frac{1}{2}$
B. $46\frac{1}{2}$	E. 43	H. $39\frac{3}{4}$	K. 71	N. $74\frac{1}{4}$
C. $45\frac{1}{2}$	F. $41\frac{3}{4}$	I. $38\frac{1}{4}$	L. $68\frac{3}{4}$	
10. A. 4 ft	D. 4 ft 10 in	G. 6 ft 2 in	J. 6 ft 6 in	M. 5 ft $1\frac{3}{4}$ in
B. 4 ft 6 in	E. 5 ft 2 in	H. 2 ft 6 in	K. 3 ft $6\frac{1}{2}$ in	N. 4 ft $7\frac{1}{4}$ in
C. 3 ft 3 in	F. 5 ft 8 in	I. 1 ft 6 in	L. 4 ft $6\frac{1}{4}$ in	O. 6 ft $1\frac{1}{2}$ in
11. A. $1\frac{3}{4}$	D. $3\frac{3}{8}$	G. $6\frac{1}{2}$	J. 9	
B. $2\frac{1}{4}$	E. 4	H. $7\frac{5}{8}$	K. $10\frac{7}{8}$	
C. $2\frac{7}{8}$	F. $5\frac{1}{4}$	I. $8\frac{1}{4}$	L. $11\frac{5}{8}$	
12. A. 12 oz	D. 2 lb	G. 3 lb 4 oz	J. 4 lb 10 oz	
B. 1 lb 2 oz	E. 2 lb 5 oz	H. 3 lb 14 oz	K. 4 lb 15 oz	
C. 1 lb 8 oz	F. 2 lb 11 oz	I. 4 lb 6 oz	L. 5 lb 3 oz	
13. A. 1/8	D. 1/2	G. 7/8	J. $6\frac{1}{2}$	M. $12\frac{3}{4}$
B. 1/4	E. 5/8	H. 1	K. $8\frac{3}{16}$	N. $11\frac{15}{16}$
C. 3/8	F. 3/4	I. $2\frac{1}{4}$	L. $10\frac{7}{16}$	O. $15\frac{5}{8}$

CHAPTER 20:2 POSITIONING A PATIENT

1. C	5. B	9. A, F	13. C	17. H
2. H	6. B	10. I, F	14. C	18. E
3. E, H	7. G	11. I	15. B	19. D, E, H
4. D	8. H	12. G	16. F	20. B, C

21. obtain instruction or read manufacturer's instructions
22. (Any 2 of the following) close door to room, draw curtains, drape or cover patient

CHAPTER 20:3 SCREENING FOR VISION PROBLEMS

1. ability to perceive and comprehend the sense of sight
2. natural daylight with no direct sunlight
3. pictures, letter *E*, alphabet
4. heights, 20, 20
5. distance the patient is from the chart
6. height of the characters the patient can read
7. 50 mm, 20 ft, 50 ft
8. myopia or nearsightedness
9. Jaeger system
10. Ishihara method
11. patient is asked to identify number printed in colored dots against a background of colored dots

12. OD: oculus dexter, or right eye
    OS: oculus sinister, or left eye
    OU: oculus uterque, or each eye; both eyes
13. defect in distant vision, or nearsightedness
14. defect in close vision, or farsightedness

CHAPTER 20:4 ASSISTING WITH PHYSICAL EXAMINATIONS

1. a. EENT: eye, ear, nose, and throat
   b. gyn: breasts, vagina, cervix, pelvic organs of female
   c. general: all areas of the body
2. detect cancer of the cervix or reproductive organs
3. a. palpation, b. percussion, c. observation, d. auscultation
4. so bladder is empty and internal organs can be felt
5. (Any 5 of the following) height/weight, vital signs, vision screening, audiometric screening, blood tests, electrocardiogram
6. a. ophthalmoscope: examine eye; b. otoscope: examine ear; c. tuning fork: test hearing acuity; d. laryngeal mirror: examine larynx, or voice box; d. percussion hammer: test tendon reflexes; f. cervical spatula (Ayer blade): obtain or scrape cells from cervix; g. rectal speculum: examine rectum; h. sigmoidoscope: examine sigmoid colon
7. alleviate fears and reassure patient
8. (Any 3 of the following) wash hands frequently, wear gloves if contact with blood or body fluids is likely, wear personal protective equipment (PPE) if splashing/spraying is likely, disinfect or sterilize any contaminated instruments or equipment

CHAPTER 20:5 ASSISTING WITH MINOR SURGERY AND SUTURE REMOVAL

1. (Any 3 of the following) removal of warts, cysts, tumors, growths, or foreign objects; suturing wounds; incision and drainage of body areas
2. removal of stitches
3. prevent infection and maintain sterility
4. a. incise, or cut, skin and tissues
   b. cut tissues
   c. compress, or clamp, blood vessels to stop bleeding or grasp tissue
   d. grasp tissue
   e. hold or draw back the lips or sides of a wound or an incision
   f. hold or support the needle while sutures are inserted
   g. remove splinters and other foreign objects from the skin and/or tissues
   h. attach surgical drapes to each other or clamp onto tissue that has been dissected
5. cleansing the surgical site with an antiseptic soap and, at times, shaving excessive hair
6. suture scissors and thumb forceps
7. to insert under suture material so stitch can be cut and removed
8. refer questions to physician
9. place in special container immediately, label, send to laboratory
10. standard precautions

CHAPTER 20:6 RECORDING AND MOUNTING AN ELECTROCARDIOGRAM

1. sinoatrial (SA) node, atria, atrioventricular (AV) node, bundle of His, right and left bundle branches, Purkinje fibers
2. a. P wave: impulse originates in SA node and travels through atria, atrial depolarization
   b. QRS: impulse moves through AV node, bundle of His, bundle branches, and Perkinje fibers, ventricular depolarization
   c. T wave: repolarization of the ventricles, period of recovery when ventricles relax

3. one
4. to determine which parts of the heart are diseased or malfunctioning
5. 12
6. RA: right arm; LL: left leg; RL: right leg; LA: left arm
7.

V_1—.	V_4—. . . .	1 .	aVR—
V_2—. .	V_5—.	2 . .	aVL— —
V_3—. . .	V_6—.	3 . . .	aVF— — —

8. single channel produces narrow strip of paper showing one lead at a time, multiple channel produces a full sheet of paper with all 12 leads
9. a. tracing light: increase stylus heat
   b. standard eight blocks high: adjust standard control
   c. complexes tiny: set sensitivity at 2
   d. complexes close together: use run 50
10. 10, 2
11. 1, 25
12. nervous tension can interfere with an accurate reading: (any 2 of the following) stress that test is not painful or uncomfortable, position patient comfortably, reassure patient

CHAPTER 20:7 ASSIGNMENT SHEET #1 USING THE *PHYSICIANS' DESK REFERENCE* (PDR)

1. 345 Park Avenue, New York, NY 10154-0037; (212) 546-4000; Internet address: www.bms.com
2. see list in PDR under alphabetical index by manufacturer
3. a. Synthroid: Abbott Laboratories; replacement of thyroid hormone for hypothyroidism; severe headache, palpitations, chest pain, diarrhea, irritability, excitability, insomnia, intolerance to heat, significant weight loss, and/or excessive sweating; usually 75 to 125 micrograms (mcg) per day but doses up to 200 mcg per day may be required
   b. Esidrex: Hydrochorothiazide; diuretic/antihypertensive; check for fluid and electrolyte imbalance, may cause glucose intolerance; respiratory distress, sensitivity reactions, electrolyte imbalance, orthostatic hypotension, anorexia, gastrointestinal disturbances, hyperglycemia, dizziness, vertigo, headache; 25–100 mg qd or bid
4. a. Metformin hydrochloride: Fortamet, Glucophage, Riomet, see list under Generic and Chemical Name Index
   b. Vitamin B_{12}: see list under Generic and Chemical Name Index
5. see lists under hemorrhoids in Product Classification Index

CHAPTER 20:7 ASSIGNMENT SHEET #2 USING THE *PHYSICIANS' DESK REFERENCE* (PDR)

1. Merck and Company, One Merck Drive, Whitehouse Station, NJ 08889; (908) 423-1000
2. a. Demerol hydrochloride: narcotic analgesic, spasmolytic, sedative; may be habit-forming; dizziness, nausea and vomiting, constipation, flushing face, dry mouth, weakness, hypotension, profuse perspiration; 50–150 mg q3–4h
   b. Erythromycin tablets: antibiotic, macrolide; nausea and vomiting, abdominal discomfort, diarrhea, sensitivity reactions, urticaria, stains developing on teeth; 250–500 mg qid for ten days
   c. Motrin: nonsteroidal anti-inflammatory, analgesic; do not take with aspirin, use with caution in people on anticoagulant therapy or with hypersensitivity, contraindicated in pregnancy; nausea, diarrhea, ulcer, abdominal pain, signs of liver damage, dizziness, headache, rash, edema, tinnitus; 200–400 mg tid or qid, dose should not exceed 1,200 mg per day
3. The Product Identification Section of the PDR
4. (Any 4 of the following) achromycin, mysteclin, Nu-Tetra, panmycin, sumycin, tetracyn
5. (Any 4 of the following) thyroid, levothroid, synthroid, thyrolar, cytomel, euthroid, proloid, liothyronine

CHAPTER 20:7 ASSIGNMENT SHEET #3 USING THE *PHYSICIANS' DESK REFERENCE* (PDR)

1. Pharmacia Corporation, 100 Route 206 North, Peapack, NJ 07977
2. see list under Pharmacia in alphabetical index by manufacturer
3. a. Vibramycin capsules: antibiotic; gastrointestinal irritation, skin rash, hypersensitive reactions, discoloration of teeth during tooth development, photosensitivity, see list in text; 100 mg qd
   b. Lanoxin: strengthens and slows cardiac activity, use for congestive heart failure, atrial fibrillation/flutter; watch for toxic effects, potassium depletion, use with caution and at reduced dosage in elderly clients, pregnant woman, nursing mothers, and newborns; 0.125–0.5 mg qd
   c. Darvon compound: narcotic analgesic; dizziness, headache, visual disturbances, sedation, skin rash, gastrointestinal disturbances; 32–65 mg q4h
4. Amoxicillin: amoxil 250 or amoxil 500; antibiotic; 500 mg q8h or q12h; yes, children over 3 months; safe use in pregnancy has not been established, but it may decrease the effectiveness of oral contraceptives
5. see list in Product Category Index under coughs and colds

CHAPTER 20:8 WORKING WITH MATH AND MEDICATIONS

1. (Any 3 of the following) aqueous suspension, suspension, syrup, tincture
2. (Any 3 of the following) capsule, pill, tablet, troche (or lozenge), enteric-coated
3. (Any 3 of the following) ointments, pastes, creams, suppositories
4. a. oral: by mouth; b. rectal: into rectum; c. subcutaneous: injected into layer of tissue just under the skin; d. intramuscular: injected into a muscle; e. intravenous: injected into a vein; f. topical: applied directly to the top of the skin; g. sublingual: given under the tongue
5. right medication, dose or amount, patient, time, method of administration, documentation
6. three (3), when taking bottle from shelf, while pouring, when replacing bottle
7. safe, cool, dry area, out of reach of children
8. throw it out
9. follow agency policy and federal and state laws; if the policies/laws call for destruction of the medications, flush them down the toilet; record all information according to agency policy
10. return to pharmacy as required by law, complete all required documentation

CHAPTER 20:8A USING ROMAN NUMERALS

1.	I	LXXII	CCCXLIII	2.	26	97	971
	VII	LXXXVIII	DX		11	122	1,150
	XI	IC or XCIX	DCXXII		9	144	1,950
	XIII	CIV	XM or CMXC		54	403	1,980
	XVIII	CX	MXV		75	456	3,000
	XXII	CXXIX	MCMLXXXVII				
	LIV	CL	MCMIC or MCMXCIX				

3.	10	25	4.	100	50
	5	30		500	100
	15	7		1,000	500
				2,000	750

CHAPTER 20:8B CONVERTING METRIC MOVEMENTS

(1)	1	0.5	(2)	2	3.5	(3)	1	0.75
	1.5	3.5		0.5	2.5		0.25	2.55
	5	0.25		1.85	0.1		4	10

(4)	5,000	3,000	(5)	2,000	100	(6)	70,000	22,300
	2,500	6,250		5,500	3,500		35,240	885,000
	10,000	8,875		10,000	7,000		1,180,000	64.32
(7)	2.28	0.2732	(8)	0.64	42	(9)	580,000	42.5
	89.21	5.40		0.00228	0.1		47,000	1,520
	0.0832	0.0023		9.8	0.0055432		381	296,000
(10)	3	4,500						
	2.5	3,250						
	5,600	5,000,000						
	0.08264	0.032						
	321.14	42.5						

CHAPTER 20:8C CONVERTING HOUSEHOLD (ENGLISH) MEASUREMENTS

(1)	10 oz	2 oz	(2)	120 mL	165 mL	(3)	3 tsp	$1\frac{1}{2}$ tsp
	8 oz	$4\frac{1}{2}$ oz		240 mL	210 mL		8 tsp	4 tsp
	30 oz	$1\frac{1}{2}$ oz		300 mL	360 mL		5 tsp	6 tsp
(4)	25 mL	50 mL	(5)	1 tbsp	2 tbsp	(6)	15 gtts	45 gtts
	10 mL	40 mL		4 tbsp	10 tbsp		75 gtts	105 gtts
	5 mL	35 mL		3 tbsp	9 tbsp		225 gtts	1,200 gtts
(7)	55.388 kg	110.322 kg	(8)	8 oz	40 oz	(9)	0.45 m	1.86 m
	94.432 kg	49.032 kg		32 oz	12 oz		0.75 m	96,096 m
	64.922 kg	41.768 kg		16 oz	8.5 oz		4.55 m	164,964.8 m
(10)	1 pt	4 qt						
	$1\frac{1}{2}$ qt	5 pt						
	3 qt	$1\frac{1}{2}$ pt						
	16 oz	18 tbsp						
	12 tsp	41 oz						

CHAPTER 21 NURSE ASSISTANT SKILLS

CHAPTER 21:1 ADMITTING, TRANSFERRING, AND DISCHARGING PATIENTS

1. anxiety, fear
2. (Any 3 of the following) by being courteous, supportive, and kind; provide clear instructions on how to operate equipment; explain the routine schedule; do not hurry or rush the patient; allow patient to ask questions and express concerns
3. relative or person responsible for patient
4. (Any 3 of the following) place in safe, description of valuables put on valuable's envelope, money left in wallet counted and recorded, both assistant and patient should check items and sign envelope, receipt for valuables given to patient
5. (Any 6 of the following) operate call signal, operate bed controls, operate television, use telephone, visiting hours, location of lounges, smoking regulations, availability of services, times for meals, other rules or routines
6. transfer because of change in patient's condition, transfer made at patient's request
7. (Any 2 of the following) clothing, personal items, equipment
8. doctor's order

9. report immediately to your supervisor
10. to ensure that all procedures have been followed
11. answers will be individualized: check the admission form to ascertain that information is complete

CHAPTER 21:2 POSITIONING, TURNING, MOVING, AND TRANSFERRING PATIENTS

1. Alignment: positioning the patient in such a way that all body parts are in proper relation to each other to maintain correct body posture
2. (Any 2 of the following) fatigue, pressure ulcers, contractures
3. two; (any 3 of the following) provides exercise for muscles, stimulates circulation, prevents pressure ulcers and contractures, provides comfort
4. tightening, or shortening, of the muscles usually caused by a lack of movement or usage of the muscle
5. bedsore, or pressure sore, caused by prolonged pressure on an area of the body that interferes with circulation
6. stage I: red or blue-gray discoloration on intact skin
   stage II: abrasions, bruises, and open sores develop
   stage III: deep open crater forms
   stage IV: damage extends into muscle, tendon, and bone tissue
7. at start, after patient is in dangling position, at end
8. determines how well patient tolerates procedure
9. (Any 5 of the following) changes in pulse rate, changes in respirations, color, weakness, dizziness, increased perspiration, discomfort
10. approval, orders, immediate supervisor, never

CHAPTER 21:3 BEDMAKING

1. wrinkles cause discomfort and can lead to pressure ulcers
2. mitered corners hold linen firmly in place
3. to welcome patient, for ambulatory patient
4. occupied bed is made while patient is in bed, closed bed is made after patient is discharged
5. a bed cradle will prevent bed linen from touching parts of the body
6. (Any 5 of the following) leg injury, blood clot, burns, skin ulcers, leg/foot surgery, circulatory disease, fractures
7. half sheets that extend from the patient's shoulders to the knees; used to protect the mattress
8. shaking spreads germs
9. saves time and energy
10. open end is away from the door, looks neater, protects against germs that enter from the hall

CHAPTER 21:4 ADMINISTERING PERSONAL HYGIENE

1. (Any 6 of the following) bath, back care, oral hygiene, hair care, nail care, shaving, shower, tub bath
2. patient is confined to bed and assistant bathes all parts of the body
3. only the face, hands, arms, back, and perineal area are bathed; patient washes parts he or she is able to wash, and assistant washes rest of the body
4. (Any 3 of the following) prevents disease, prevents caries, stimulates the appetite, provides comfort, prevents halitosis
5. unconscious or semiconscious patient
6. (Any 3 of the following) stimulates circulation to scalp, prevents scalp disease, removes dirt and/or lint, helps keep the hair shiny and attractive
7. nails harbor dirt and can lead to infection, rough or sharp nails can cause injury
8. nail clippers, scissors, straight across, tips
9. injuries to the feet are prone to infection and slow to heal
10. regular or electric razors, patient's personal preference

11. stimulates circulation, prevents pressure ulcers, leads to relaxation and comfort
12. remove sleeve from unaffected arm first, then from injured arm or arm with IV
13. (Any 5 of the following) sores, cuts, injuries, rash, color, swelling (or edema), dyspnea, vertigo, unusual weakness, diaphoresis, extreme pallor, lethargy
14. a. erythema: redness, b. cyanosis: blue color, c. jaundice: yellow color, d. vertigo: dizziness, e. dyspnea: difficult breathing, f. diaphoresis: excessive perspiration (or sweating), g. lethargy: excessive drowsiness or sluggishness
15. (Any 3 of the following) wash hands frequently, wear gloves if contact with blood or body fluids is likely, wear gowns if contamination of uniform or clothing is likely, wear masks and protective eyewear if droplets of blood or body fluids are present
16. (Any 3 of the following) knock on door and pause before entering, close door, screen unit, avoid exposing patient during procedure
17. answers will be individualized but should include:
    a. report rash immediately
    b. report to supervisor and obtain an order for shampooing
    c. explain reason for electric razor; if Mr. Mollica refuses shave, check with supervisor
    d. leave the gown in place and report this to the supervisor immediately
    e. turn him back over and call for your supervisor

CHAPTER 21:5A MEASURING AND RECORDING INTAKE AND OUTPUT

Instructor: Set up a station with measuring devices listed on the assignment sheet so students can practice measuring with metric units. Measurements will vary slightly, but answers should be close to those listed.

(1) 5 mL 15 mL	(2) 4 oz 120 mL	(3) 8 oz 240 mL	(4) 12 or 14 oz 360 or 420 mL	(5) 8 oz 240 mL
(6) 6 oz 180 mL	(7) 11 oz or 12 oz 330 mL or 360 mL	(8) 1 cup 8 oz 240 mL	(9) 32 oz 4 cup 2 pint 1 quart 1,000 mL	(10) 16 c 8 pt 4 qt 128 oz 4,000 mL
(11) 2 c 1 pt 16 oz 500 mL	(12) 450 gtts 2 tbsp 1 oz 30 mL			

CHAPTER 21:5B RECORDING INTAKE AND OUTPUT #1

Assignment No. 1 (of 21:5B)

INTAKE AND OUTPUT RECORD

Family Name	First Name	Attending Physician	Room No.	Hosp. No.
JONES	SAM	DR. MARANDEZ	236	

Date	INTAKE				OUTPUT					OTHER				REMARKS
TIME	Oral	I.V.	Blood		Urine	Tube	Emesis	Feces						
7–8 a.m.														
8–9 a.m.	600													
9–10 a.m.					400									
10–11 a.m.														
11–12 noon	680													
12–1 p.m.	180													
1–2 p.m.					550									1 FORMED BM
2–3 p.m.	180	800												
8-HOUR TOTAL	1640	800			950									
3–4 p.m.														
4–5 p.m.							550							EMESIS—DXGREEN
5–6 p.m.	220													
6–7 p.m.	240													
7–8 p.m.														
8–9 p.m.					480									
9–10 p.m.														
10–11 p.m.	180	750												
8-HOUR TOTAL	640	750			480		550							
11–12 p.m.														
12–1 a.m.														
1–2 a.m.														
2–3 a.m.	180													
3–4 a.m.														
4–5 a.m.					550			300						BM—LT. BROWN LIQUID
5–6 a.m.														
6–7 a.m.	180	850												
8-HOUR TOTAL	360	850			550			300						
24 HOUR TOTAL	2640	2400			1980		550	300						
	TOTAL INTAKE 5040				TOTAL OUTPUT 2830									

CHAPTER 21:5B RECORDING INTAKE AND OUTPUT #2

Assignment No. 2 (of 21:5B)

INTAKE AND OUTPUT RECORD

Family Name	First Name	Attending Physician	Room No.	Hosp. No.
WRAY	FRED	DR. PEASE	2851	

Date	INTAKE				OUTPUT					OTHER				REMARKS
TIME	Oral	I.V.	Blood	N/G	Urine	Tube	Emesis	Feces						
7–8 a.m.	10			20	30									NG IRR: NS
8–9 a.m.	15				40									
9–10 a.m.	5				25									
10–11 a.m.					30									
11–12 noon	15				35									NG IRR: NS
12–1 p.m.	15			30	40									
1–2 p.m.	15				25		100							EMESIS.CL LIQUID
2–3 p.m.		1000			25	750								NG: GREENISH
8-HOUR TOTAL	75	1000		50	250	750	100							
3–4 p.m.	10				15									
4–5 p.m.				10	30									NG IRR: NS
5–6 p.m.	15				10									
6–7 p.m.					20									
7–8 p.m.	10				40									
8–9 p.m.				20	30									NG IRR: NS
9–10 p.m.					25									
10–11 p.m.	15	950			30	990								NG: GREENISH
8-HOUR TOTAL	50	950		30	200	990								
11–12 p.m.					10									NG IRR: NS
12–1 a.m.	15			20	0									
1–2 a.m.	15				5									
2–3 a.m.				10	5									NG IRR: NS
3–4 a.m.	15				0									
4–5 a.m.	10			10	10									NG IRR: NS
5–6 a.m.	15				15									
6–7 a.m.		1050		10	20	650								NG: GOLDEN NG IRR: NS
8-HOUR TOTAL	70	1050		50	65	650								
24 HOUR TOTAL	195	3000		130	515	2390	100							
	TOTAL INTAKE 3325				TOTAL OUTPUT 3005									

CHAPTER 21:5B RECORDING INTAKE AND OUTPUT #3

Assignment No. 3 (of 21:5B)

INTAKE AND OUTPUT RECORD

Family Name: PERRY First Name: TAMIKA Attending Physician: DR. KOWALSKI Room No. Hosp. No.

Date	INTAKE				OUTPUT					OTHER				REMARKS
TIME	Oral	I.V.	Blood	N/G	Urine	Tube	Emesis	Feces						
7–8 a.m.	10			10										NG IRR: NS
8–9 a.m.	30													
9–10 a.m.	60				400									
10–11 a.m.														
11–12 noon	120			10				300						BM: GREENISH NG IRR: NS
12–1 p.m.	10	400												
1–2 p.m.	15				250									
2–3 p.m.		150				780	100							NG: GREENISH EMESIS: CL LIQUID
8-HOUR TOTAL	245	550		20	650	780	100	300						
3–4 p.m.														
4–5 p.m.	10			10										NG IRR: NS
5–6 p.m.	45				375			200						BM: GREENISH
6–7 p.m.	120													
7–8 p.m.														
8–9 p.m.	30	500												
9–10 p.m.				15	550		130							EMESIS: REDDISH BROWN NG IRR: NS
10–11 p.m.	10	200				550								NG: GOLDEN BROWN
8-HOUR TOTAL	215	700		25	925	550	130	200						
11–12 p.m.														
12–1 a.m.	30													
1–2 a.m.	60			10	400									NG IRR: NS
2–3 a.m.	10													
3–4 a.m.	15	400						750						BM: GREENISH
4–5 a.m.	90			15										NG IRR: NS
5–6 a.m.					200		200							EMESIS: GOLDEN GREEN
6–7 a.m.		200				625								NG: GOLDEN BROWN
8-HOUR TOTAL	205	600		25	600	625	200	750						
24 HOUR TOTAL	665	1850		70	2175	1955	430	1250						
	TOTAL INTAKE 2585				TOTAL OUTPUT 5810									

CHAPTER 21:5B RECORDING INTAKE AND OUTPUT #4

Assignment No. 4 (of 21:5B)

INTAKE AND OUTPUT RECORD

Family Name	First Name	Attending Physician	Room No.	Hosp. No.
WRECKLESS	JOHN	DR. SANTORO	1835	

Date	INTAKE				OUTPUT					OTHER				REMARKS
TIME	Oral	I.V.	Blood	N/G	Urine	Tube	Emesis	Feces						
7–8 a.m.	90													
8–9 a.m.	300													
9–10 a.m.	5													
10–11 a.m.	120		500	10	800									NG IRR: NS IV: BLOOD
11–12 noon	10						200							EMESIS: CL LIQUID
12–1 p.m.	280													
1–2 p.m.	5	400		15		20								NG IRR: NS HEMOVAC: REDDISH
2–3 p.m.	120	500			600	800								NG: REDDISH BROWN
8-HOUR TOTAL	930	900	500	25	1400	820	200							
3–4 p.m.	5													
4–5 p.m.	90 10							300						BM: LT BROWN
5–6 p.m.	300			10										NG IRR: NS
6–7 p.m.	120													
7–8 p.m.	5													
8–9 p.m.	120	100												
9–10 p.m.	120			10		15								NG IRR: NS HEMOVAC: PINK
10–11 p.m.	10	600			940	750								NG: GOLDEN BROWN
8-HOUR TOTAL	780	700		20	940	765		300						
11–12 p.m.								250						BM: LT BROWN
12–1 a.m.	90			15										NG IRR: NS
1–2 a.m.														
2–3 a.m.	5		500		850									IV: PLASMA
3–4 a.m.	120						350							EMESIS: GREENISH
4–5 a.m.	10			10										NG IRR: NS
5–6 a.m.	120	600		15		10								NG IRR: NS HEMOVAC: PINK
6–7 a.m.		200			160	400								NG: GREENISH
8-HOUR TOTAL	345	800	500	40	1010	410	350	250						
24-HOUR TOTAL	2055	2400	1000	85	3350	1995	550	550						
	TOTAL INTAKE		5540		TOTAL OUTPUT			6445						

CHAPTER 21:5B RECORDING INTAKE AND OUTPUT #5

Assignment No. 5 (of 21:5B)

INTAKE AND OUTPUT RECORD

Family Name	First Name	Attending Physician	Room No.	Hosp. No.
O'CONNOR	MARANDA	DR. SCHMIDT	ICU	

Date	INTAKE				OUTPUT					OTHER				REMARKS
TIME	Oral	I.V.	Blood	N/G	Urine	Tube	Emesis	Feces						
7–8 a.m.	90													
8–9 a.m.	300													1 FORMED STOOL
9–10 a.m.	5						200							EMESIS: CL LIQUID
10–11 a.m.	120	200		10	400									NG IRR: NS
11–12 noon	5													
12–1 p.m.	10 680													
1–2 p.m.	90			10	550									NG IRR: NS
2–3 p.m.	15	550				550								NG: GREENISH BROWN
8-HOUR TOTAL	1315	750		20	950	550	200							
3–4 p.m.	5													
4–5 p.m.	10													
5–6 p.m.	15 440			15	400									NG IRR: NS
6–7 p.m.	90													
7–8 p.m.	120						300	200						EMESIS: BROWNISH BM: BROWN LIQUID
8–9 p.m.		450												
9–10 p.m.	90			10										NG IRR: NS
10–11 p.m.	5	100			qs	200								PT. INCONTINENT NG: GOLDEN BROWN
8-HOUR TOTAL	775	550		25	400+	200	300	200						
11–12 p.m.														
12–1 a.m.	10													
1–2 a.m.	180				500									
2–3 a.m.	10	100		10				300						NG IRR: NS BM: BROWN LIQ
3–4 a.m.														
4–5 a.m.					650									
5–6 a.m.	180			10										NG IRR: NS
6–7 a.m.		200				450								NG: GREENISH
8-HOUR TOTAL	380	300		20	1150	450		300						
24-HOUR TOTAL	2470	1600		65	2500+	1200	500	500						
	TOTAL INTAKE			4135	TOTAL OUTPUT			4700+						

CHAPTER 21:6 FEEDING A PATIENT

1. offer bedpan or urinal, wash hands and face, position in sitting position, provide oral hygiene if desired, clear overbed table, remove unpleasant objects
2. explain this fact to the patient
3. check with immediate supervisor or dietitian
4. check with immediate supervisor or dietitian to see if a substitute can be provided
5. (Any 3 of the following) name, room number, type of diet, food on the tray
6. compare plate of food to a clock and tell patient the location of each item, arrange utensils conveniently
7. place small amount on wrist
8. (Any 3 of the following) alternate liquids and solids, use straws for liquids, hold utensils at right angle to mouth, encourage patient to eat as much as possible; provide relaxed, unhurried atmosphere; give patient sufficient time to chew
9. keep a record of nutritional intake
10. (Any 2 of the following) feed small quantities, allow patient time to chew and swallow, provide liquids to keep mouth moist

CHAPTER 21:7 ASSISTING WITH A BEDPAN/URINAL

1. emptying of the bladder; discharge of waste through rectum
2. death would be the result
3. fracture or orthopedic, standard bedpan
4. (Any 2 of the following) close door, close privacy curtain, close window curtain
5. (Any 3 of the following) frequency, amount, appearance, abnormalities
6. intake and output, measured, recorded
7. report it immediately, save a specimen
8. sensitive, privacy, comfortable, immediately
9. (Any 5 of the following) wash hands frequently, wear gloves, wear eye protection if splashing/spraying is possible, disinfect bedpan or urinal after use, use bedpan or urinal for one patient and sterilize before using for another patient, wipe contaminated areas with disinfectants, allow patient to wash hands and receive perineal care
10. protect environmental surfaces from contamination with substances on gloved hands

CHAPTER 21:8 PROVIDING CATHETER AND URINARY-DRAINAGE UNIT CARE

1. catheters
2. balloon, sterile water, the catheter in place
3. (Any 6 of the following) connection between catheter and unit is secure; tubing is free from kinks or bends, drainage bag is below level of bladder; urine is flowing freely; catheter is taped, strapped, or tied to leg; drainage unit is emptied frequently; drainage bag is attached to bed frame; no loops of drainage tube are below bag; drainage tube in bag is above level of urine; any patient complaints of burning, pain, irritation, or tenderness in the urethral area
4. backflow of urine into bladder, could cause infection
5. use special urine collection area on tubing if available or disconnect catheter from unit
6. prevent infection
7. keep urinary meatus clean and free of secretions to help prevent bladder and kidney infections
8. (Any 3 of the following) amount, color, type, presence of other substances
9. report immediately
10. develop voluntary control of urination and prevent incontinence

CHAPTER 21:9 PROVIDING OSTOMY CARE

1. surgical procedure in which an opening called a stoma is created in the abdominal wall
2. (Any 4 of the following) tumors and/or cancer, birth defects, ulcerative colitis, bowel obstructions, injuries
3. a. ureterostomy, b. colostomy, c. ileostomy

4. stool from ascending colostomy is more liquid, whereas stool from sigmoid colostomy is similar to normal stool; water and other substances have been reabsorbed when stool reaches sigmoid colon
5. leakage, odor, irritation of the skin surrounding the stoma
6. prevent irritation from the removal of the pouch; (any 3 of the following) wafers, pastes, powders, liquid films
7. allow patient to express feelings and verbalize fears, provide understanding and support
8. bright to dark red in color with wet appearance
9. a. low hemoglobin level, b. dehydration, c. interference with blood supply
10. amount, color, type of discharge

CHAPTER 21:10 COLLECTING STOOL/URINE SPECIMENS

1. urine is more concentrated and may reveal more abnormalities, acid pH preserves any cells present
2. 120, send amount available
3. refrigerate specimen
4. obtain specimen free from contamination
5. female: front to back motion, external lips, then internal lips, then center
   male: circular motion from meatus down
6. sterile container and lid
7. catherize patient
8. it was produced before the start of the test
9. chemicals, cold storage
10. to keep at body temperature, and examine within 30 minutes for most accurate results
11. blood is present in the stool
12. to avoid contamination from spills

CHAPTER 21:11 GIVING ENEMAS AND RECTAL TREATMENTS

1. injection of fluid into the large intestine through the rectum
2. (Any 2 of the following) remove feces and flatus, relieve intestinal congestion, give medication
3. retention: kept in intestine for specified period of time
   nonretention: expelled in 5–10 minutes, usually given in larger quantities
4. a cleansing: remove stool and flatus
   b. disposable: stimulate peristalsis
   c. oil: soften feces
5. Sims', encourages solution to flow from rectum to sigmoid colon
6. (Any 3 of the following) amount, type of stool, color, amount of flatus
7. large mass of fecal material lodged in rectum: give oil-retention enema to soften impaction so it can be expelled; if enema does not remove impaction, insert gloved finger into rectum to break up fecal material
8. aid in expulsion of flatus
9. cone-shaped object with cocoa butter or glycerine base
10. (Any 3 of the following) stimulate peristalsis and expel feces, relieve pain, decrease body temperature, stop vomiting, administer medication

CHAPTER 21:12 APPLYING RESTRAINTS

1. protective devices that limit a patient's movements
2. (Any 4 of the following) behavior must be documented, alternatives must be tried, resident or guardian must give written consent, physician must write order, least restrictive device must be used first
3. (Any 3 of the following) type of restraint, reason for its use, length of time it can be used, where or when it can be used
4. irrational or confused, skin conditions, paralysis or limited muscular coordination

5. (Any 3 of the following) straps or belts: hold patient in stretcher or wheelchair; limb: limit movement of arms or legs; hand mitts: applied to hands to prevent patient from scratching or injuring skin; jacket: prevent patient from sitting up, rolling, or getting out of bed or wheelchair
6. slip two fingers between the restraint and the skin
7. (Any 5 of the following) paleness, cyanosis, cold skin, edema, weak or absent pulse, poor return of pink color after nail beds are blanched, complaints of pain/numbness/tingling
8. two, ten, repositioned, range-of-motion, skin
9. physical and mental frustration; impaired circulation; pressure ulcers; loss of muscle tone, joint stiffness, and discomfort from immobility; respiratory, or breathing, problems
10. whether the risk of potential injury to the patient or others is greater than the risk of complications from the use of restraints

CHAPTER 21:13 ADMINISTERING PRE- AND POSTOPERATIVE CARE

1. preoperative, operative, postoperative
2. (Any 10 of the following) operative permit signed, laboratory tests, enemas, vaginal irrigations, baths, skin preparation, vital signs, NPO, valuables in safe, prosthetics removed, cosmetics removed, clothing removed, check name band, voiding, surgical checklist
3. remove as many microorganisms as possible to prevent infection
4. tape or tie to the finger
5. prevent infection in and around the surgical site, remove longer hairs that would interfere with the surgery
6. follow agency policy or doctor's order
7. a. general: given by mask or IV, patient unconscious
   b. local: injected into area around op site, stops sensation
   c. spinal: injected into spinal canal, loss of sensation in all areas below injection
8. nausea and/or vomiting
9. vital signs equipment, IV stand, emesis basin, tissues, special equipment
10. (Any 6 of the following) vitals signs; check dressings; check IV; assess level of pain; observe restlessness, color of skin, nausea and/or vomiting, temperature of skin; change position; cough and breathe deeply; check drainage tubes
11. analgesic or pain medication injection into an intravenous line by an analgesic pump; patient can push button when feeling pain to obtain immediate relief
12. (Any 3 of the following) tubes not draining, tubes clamped, drainage solution changes or seems unusual, tube not connected to a drainage source, unusual observations
13. support veins of legs and increase circulation
14. special adhesive strips that are applied when dressings must be changed frequently, prevents need to remove and reapply adhesive tape during each dressing change

CHAPTER 21:14 APPLYING BINDERS

1. (Any 5 of the following) provide support, provide relief from pain, hold dressings in place, provide support for engorged breasts, limit motion, apply pressure to specific body parts
2. smoothly, pressure areas, pressure ulcers, wrinkles, creases, snug, tight
3. abdomen, back, rib cage
4. two (2)
5. make darts to ease excess material
6. support breasts especially after childbirth
7. scrotal support for men, self-adhesive sanitary napkins for women
8. bottom, top
9. circulation, breathing
10. give skin care to area under binder

CHAPTER 21:15 ADMINISTERING OXYGEN

1. some states prohibit administration of oxygen by a health care assistant
2. deficiency of oxygen
3. (Any 3 of the following) cyanosis, rapid and shallow respirations, rapid pulse, restlessness
4. mask: 6–10 liters; cannula: 2–6 liters; catheter, 2–6 liters; tent: 10–12 liters
5. a device that removes impurities and other gases from room air to concentrate oxygen in the unit; provides low liter flows of oxygen
6. oxygen is drying and can damage or irritate mucous membranes
7. (Any 4 of the following) avoid smoking, avoid open flames, place warning labels on door or tanks, avoid electrically operated equipment, do not use flammable liquids, use cotton blankets, inspect area frequently
8. level of oxygen in arterial blood
9. (Any 3 of the following) quality of respirations, mouth and nose care, rate of flow, water in humidifier, check safety precautions
10. respiratory therapy department

CHAPTER 21:16 GIVING POSTMORTEM CARE

1. care given to the body immediately after death
2. grief, loss, crying, embarrassed, emotions, support
3. (Any 4 of the following) position naturally with limbs straight, return dentures to mouth, keep bed linen neat and clean, remove extra equipment from unit, provide privacy
4. rights, dignity, respect, privacy
5. (Any 6 of the following) shroud or body bag, gown, chin strap, pads, gauze squares, ties, two or three tags, safety pins
6. remove from body, list on valuable's list, place in safe, tape wedding ring and note on chart
7. tape in place and note on chart
8. nurse or other authorized person

CHAPTER 22 PHYSICAL THERAPY SKILLS

CHAPTER 22:1 PERFORMING RANGE-OF-MOTION (ROM) EXERCISES

A: Short Answer

1. maintain health of musculoskeletal system
2. physical therapist, nurse, health care assistant, other authorized person
3. (Any 6 of the following) contractures, atrophy of muscles, poor circulation, pressure ulcers, mineral loss, brittle bones that fracture easily, renal calculi, poor appetite, constipation, urinary infections, respiratory problems, hypostatic pneumonia
4. a. active: patient moves each joint without assistance
   b. active assistive: patient moves each joint but receives assistance to complete the ROM
   c. passive: another person moves each joint for a patient who is not able to exercise
   d. resistive: exercises performed against resistance provided by a therapist
5. physical therapists, registered nurses, head, neck, hip, knee
6. part above and below joint being exercised
7. three to five times or as ordered
8. stop the exercise and report to immediate supervisor
9. expose only area being exercised, close door and screen unit

Part B: Matching

1. G	5. B	9. P	13. A	17. F
2. L	6. C	10. O	14. N	18. H
3. M	7. H	11. I	15. A	19. D
4. E	8. F	12. K	16. G	20. J

CHAPTER 22:2 AMBULATING PATIENTS WHO USE TRANSFER (GAIT) BELTS, CRUTCHES, CANES, OR WALKERS

1. underhand grasp, more secure, and hands are less likely to slip off the belt
2. a. axillary crutches; b. platform crutches; c. forearm or Lofstrand crutches
3. 1 to $1^{1}/_{2}$ inches; 4 to 6 inches; 2; 25–30 degrees
4. four-point, two-point, swing-to, swing-through
5. three-point, swing-to, swing-through
6. can injure axillary blood vessels and nerves
7. unaffected (good) side
8. 6 to 8 inches, top of femur at the hip joint, 25–30 degree angle
9. the walker may move away from the patient, causing the patient to fall
10. patients must be strong enough to hold themselves upright while leaning on a walker
11. top of femur at the hip joint, 25–30 degree angle
12. to prevent slipping
13. dangerous and easy to upset the walker while using a sliding technique
14. keep a firm hold on the transfer belt, use your body to brace the patient, ease the patient to the floor as slowly as possible while protecting the patient's head and neck, stay with the patient and call for help

CHAPTER 22:3 ADMINISTERING HEAT/COLD APPLICATIONS

1. use of cold for treatment
2. use of heat for treatment
3. vasodilation; blood vessels become larger, and more blood comes to area
4. vasoconstriction; blood vessels become smaller, and less blood comes to area
5. (Any 3 of the following) relieve pain, reduce swelling, reduce body temperature, control bleeding
6. (Any 3 of the following) relieve pain, increase drainage from an infected area, stimulate healing, increase circulation, combat infection, relieve muscle spasms, increase muscle mobility before exercise
7. a. moist cold: applications wet and cold against skin; (any 2 of the following) cold compresses, packs, or soaks
   b. dry cold: applications dry but cold against skin; (any 2 of the following) ice bags, ice collars, hypothermia blankets
   c. moist heat: applications wet and warm against skin; (any 2 of the following) sitz baths, hot soaks, compresses, hydrocollator packs, paraffin wax treatment
   d. dry heat: applications dry and warm against skin; (any 2 of the following) warm water bags, heating pads, thermal blankets, aquamatic or aquathermia pads, heat lamps
8. provide warm, moist heat to perineal and rectal areas
9. gel-filled packs warmed in a water bath
10. chronic joint disease (arthritis), ROM exercises
11. prevent the spread of infection
12. a control unit on the aquathermia pad maintains a constant preset temperature of the water
13. physician's
14. health care assistants are not allowed to administer heat or cold applications in some states and agencies
15. (Any 3 of the following) color and temperature of skin, pain, bleeding, circulation
16. metal readily conducts heat or cold and can cause injury to the skin

CHAPTER 23 BUSINESS AND ACCOUNTING SKILLS

CHAPTER 23:1A FILING RECORDS

1. systematic or orderly arrangement of papers, cards, or other materials so they are readily available for future reference
2. locate material quickly, store safely and protect as legal records
3. a. in alphabetical order following same rules used in telephone book; b. in numerical order after assigning each record a number; c. according to location, either cities, states, or countries; d. by subject or topic that the record pertains to
4. the Health Insurance Portability and Accountability Act (HIPPA) prohibits placing identifiable information such as social security numbers on the outside of a patient's chart; helps prevent identify theft if an unauthorized person should happen to see the chart
5. avoid misplaced or lost records
6. on index cards in a separate file, on colored paper placed in a file folder
7. folders are marked with series of colors in addition to name to provide a second means of verifying placement
8. different color chart stands out immediately
9. durable, quality, conveniently, fireproof, locks, packed tightly in drawers or shelves
10. active currently being used, inactive for patient who has not been seen for a number of years, closed for a patient who has died or a file that is no longer required
11. shredded or burned
12. in the hard drive or in magnetic tape reels, disks, or CDs

CHAPTER 23:1B ASSIGNMENT #1 FILING RECORDS USING THE ALPHABETICAL OR NUMERICAL SYSTEM

	Group 1: Indexing Order	Filing Order
(1)	Brown, Mary K.	Bell, Arlet Ann
	Smith, June J.	Brown, Mary K.
	Stanton, Betty M.	James, C.M.
	Thomas, Jesse Tom	Jones, Mary S.
	Bell, Arlet Ann	Smith, June J.
	James, C.M.	Stanton, Betty M.
	Jones, Mary S.	Thomas, Jesse Tom

Group 2: Indexing Order	Filing Order
Barr, A.	Barr, A.
Barr, David B., Jr	Barr, Arnold
Barr, Bruce Arnold	Barr, B.D.
Barr, B.D.	Barr, Bruce
Barr, Bruce A.	Barr, Bruce A.
Barr, Arnold	Barr, Bruce Arnold
Barr, David B., Sr	Barr, David B., Jr
Barr, Bruce	Barr, David B., Sr

Group 3: Indexing Order	Filing Order
Macerow, Cynthia	DuBarry, Mary
O'Rouge, Michael M.	Ducan, Mary D.
MacDanner, Camelia	MacDanner, Camelia
McDavis, Carol	Macer, Charles M.
O'Brian, Carl M.	Macerow, Cynthia
DuBarry, Mary	Mack, Christopher C.
Macer, Charles M.	McDavis, Carol
McDowell, Clair C.	McDowell, Clair C.

Mack, Christopher C.
Ducan, Mary D.
Mt. John, Mack M.
Mount-Smith, Jean

Mt. John, Mack M.
Mount-Smith, Jean
O'Brian, Carl M.
O'Rouge, Michael M.

Group 4: Indexing Order
Kirk, Carl (Clinton, Iowa)
Kirk, Carol
Kirk, Carl (Ashland, Ohio)
Kirk, C.
Kirk, Harry (RN) (Ash, Ohio)
Krirk, Genevieve
Krickey, Roger
Mounts, Michael
McKirk, Lanna
Mt. Kirk, Mike
Kirk, Harry (MD) (Bath, Ohio)
Kirk, Harry (DDS) (Sandusky, Ohio)

Filing Order
Kirk, C.
Kirk, Carl (Clinton, Iowa)
Kirk, Carl (Ashland, Ohio)
Kirk, Carol
Kirk, Harry (RN) (Ash, Ohio)
Kirk, Harry (MD) (Bath, Ohio)
Kirk, Harry (DDS) (Sandusky, Ohio)
Krickey, Roger
Krirk, Genevieve
McKirk, Lanna
Mt. Kirk, Mike
Mounts, Michael

(2)
00034
0039
0086
249
00250
288
00289
456
588
0987
5678
9870

(3)

System 1	*System 2*
02-34-88	00-94-90
04-66-88	03-94-90
06-76-88	05-65-90
22-43-88	06-82-90
24-32-88	07-77-90
45-34-88	08-99-90
52-45-88	34-33-90
55-34-88	43-42-90
62-62-88	45-33-90
62-66-88	70-67-90

CHAPTER 23:1B ASSIGNMENT #2 FILING RECORDS USING THE ALPHABETICAL OR NUMERICAL SYSTEM

(1) **Group 1: Indexing Order**
Sainer, Judy
St. John, Stacy
Stacy, John S.
Stadler, Jill
St. Clair, Joseph
Scott, Michael
Scanlon, Lois
Scodova, Bob
Set, Frederick C.
Sanborn, Mike M.
Stanton, John
Sanborn, Mike

Filing Order
Sainer, Judy
St. Clair, Joseph
St. John, Stacy
Sanborn, Mike
Sanborn, Mike M.
Scanlon, Lois
Scodova, Bob
Scott, Michael
Set, Frederick C.
Stacy, John S.
Stadler, Jill
Stanton, John

Group 2: Indexing Order

Russ, Henry
Rush, Tom E., Jr
Rush, Rupert C.
Rusk, Herbert
Russ, Henry C.
Rush, Orville D.
Rush, Tom D., Sr
Rusell, Robert A.
Russell, Barbara D.
Rush, Tom Dean, Jr
Rurals, Michael
Rusiska, Brent T.
Russell, Bonnie F.
Russel, Kenneth K.
Ruster, Lennie L.
Rustert, Mabel M.
Rusher, Florence C.
O'Rush, Connie S.
Russell-Brown, Mary

Filing Order

O'Rush, Connie S.
Rurals, Michael
Rusell, Robert A.
Rush, Orville D.
Rush, Rupert C.
Rush, Tom D., Sr
Rush, Tom E., Jr
Rush, Tom Dean, Jr
Rusher, Florence C.
Rusiska, Brent T.
Rusk, Herbert
Russ, Henry
Russ, Henry C.
Russel, Kenneth K.
Russell, Barbara D.
Russell, Bonnie F.
Russell-Brown, Mary
Ruster, Lennie L.
Rustert, Mabel M.

Group 3: Indexing Order

Third, Street, Ambulance, Supplies
EMS, Supply, Corporation
Fourth, Street, Medical, Supplies
Smith, Mike, (DDS) (Miami, Florida)
American, Medical, Association
American, Nurses, Association
Albian, A., M., Company
Dr., John's, Foot, Pads
Smith, Mike, (MD) (Lakeland, Florida)
Smith, Mike, A. (ATR) (Arcadia, Florida)
Company (The), Medical (For), Supplies
Smith, M., A., Pharmacy
Smith, Medical, Equipment, Miami (of), Florida
Second, Avenue, Pharmacy

Filing Order

Albian, A., M., Company
American, Medical, Association
American, Nurses, Association
Company (The), Medical (for), Supplies
Dr., John's, Foot, Pads
EMS, Supply, Corporation
Fourth, Street, Medical, Supplies
Second, Avenue, Pharmacy
Smith, M., A., Pharmacy
Smith, Medical, Equipment, Miami (of), Florida
Smith, Mike, (MD) (Lakeland, Florida)
Smith, Mike, (DDS) (Miami, Florida)
Smith, Mike, A., (ATR) (Arcadia, Florida)
Third, Street, Ambulance, Supplies

(2)

0005	555
008	00555
50	0567
0058	0582
0062	0850
080	05820
082	005821
0085	5822
00088	85200

(3)

System 1	*System 2*
0002-65	0002-77
0020-65	0020-77
0033-65	0200-77
0324-65	3891-77
0333-65	4004-77
2435-65	4328-77
3245-65	4657-77
3333-65	5682-77
3425-65	5862-77
4328-65	5865-77

CHAPTER 23:2 USING THE TELEPHONE

1. (Any 4 of the following) pleasant, low-pitched, clear, distinct, no monotone or indifferent tone
2. promptly, smile
3. (Any 5 of the following) name of caller, telephone number, message, date, time of call, action taken, initials
4. a. Hello, Dr. _____'s office, Ms. _____ speaking
   b. May I have your name please?
   c. May I tell Dr. _____ why you are calling?
   d. Would you please repeat your name?
   e. The doctor is not available at present.
   f. Would you please repeat that?
   g. The doctor will not take calls unless I tell him/her who is calling.
   h. If you will leave your name and telephone number, I will give the doctor the message.
   i. Thank you for calling. Good-bye.
   j. The doctor is busy at present. May I have your telephone number so he/she can call you back?
5. avoid disturbing the doctor for calls that can be handled by another worker in the office
6. name of caller, purpose of call
7. process of evaluating the situation and prioritizing treatment
8. if you hang up first, you might miss something the caller wanted to say
9. allows a large number of telephone calls to be answered at the same time
10. allows two-way communication in almost any location, individual does not have to use another telephone to respond
11. other people can hear the cellular signal by using a scanner
12. yes; if sent on a secure Internet network; no, if sent on an insecure Internet network because it can be intercepted and read by others
13. (Any 5 of the following) have patient's written authorization, never fax financial information, fax only to machines in secure locations, use a cover sheet that contains a confidentiality statement, use a patient reference number instead of the patient's name, contact receiver before faxing, check with receiver after information is faxed, mail records or send with messenger if in doubt
14. Examples of messages: (these will vary)
   a. Dr. Jones
      Mrs. Smith
      522-5409
      Daughter Melinda has fever of 102°. No other symptoms.
      Can bring in at four o'clock or call in prescription
   b. Dr. Jones
      Dr. Peterson
      See below
      Has findings on Mrs. Complaint
      1–4 PM at office 528-0991
      4–6 PM at hospital 524-2118 ext. 34
      after 7 at home 756-6677
   c. Dr. Jones
      John Cauffwell, Ace Medical
      (442) 560-4560 ext. 110
      ECG paper 524 no longer available. New substitute 529 more expensive. Both equal quality. Can locate old stock or send new paper
   d. Dr. Jones
      Hospital—Mrs. Efficient—ward 5B
      524-2118, ext. 5566
      Johnny Pothman vomited bright red blood at 9:40 AM
      CALL STAT
   e. review messages to be sure information is concise, words are spelled correctly, and information is printed clearly
   f. #1 would be d; #2, a; #3, b; #4, c

UNIT 23:3 ASSIGNMENT SHEET #1 SCHEDULING APPOINTMENTS

Time	MONDAY	TUESDAY
8:00	Maddie East (Mike)—shot, 756-1824	
8:15		
8:30		
8:45		
9:00	Carol Bjore (Chuck)—589-2897	Beth Wilfong (Randy) Pap—522-0689
9:15	wart removal foot	Sue Hockensmith (Ray)—524-9964
9:30	Melody Jett—laryngitis—524-9293	allergy tests
9:45	Tami Conery (Scott)—797-6116	Kim Staup (Dave) cold—522-2321
10:00	ingrown toenail	Ann Henegar—physical—756-1184
10:15		
10:30	Lisa Haumesser—ear inf.—522-7723	
10:45	Chris Frey—524-8713	
11:00	growth—rt. arm	Sandy Riggenbach—797-2418
11:15		physical
11:30		
11:45		
12:00		
12:15	(lunch)	(lunch)
12:30		
12:45		
1:00	Frieda Shade (Randy)—522-8680	
1:15	Ron, Bob, Bozo, immun.	
1:30	Jim Johnson—X- ray arm—589-3156	Medical Board Meeting
1:45	Robert Hephner—Allergy sh.—589-8152	
2:00	Debbie Hillborn (Terry)—589-0302	
2:15	children—colds	
2:30		
2:45		
3:00	Diana Fletcher—797-5433	Nellie Smith (John)—589-2008
3:15	physical	physical
3:30		
3:45		
4:00	Debbie Koppert—522-5564	Duane Yoder—589-0020
4:15	stomach	X -ray chest
4:30		

UNIT 23:3 ASSIGNMENT SHEET #2 SCHEDULING APPOINTMENTS

WEDNESDAY	
8:00	
8:15	
8:30	
8:45	
9:00	Jill Johnson (Mike)—589-7191
9:15	wart removal
9:30	
9:45	
10:00	
10:15	
10:30	Chris Bell—burn arm—522-1948
10:45	Cindy Gross (Mike)—525-1149
11:00	physical
11:15	
11:30	
11:45	Tina Shepher—knee—886-7022
12:00	
12:15	(lunch)
12:30	
12:45	
1:00	Dental Appointment
1:15	
1:30	
1:45	
2:00	
2:15	
2:30	
2:45	
3:00	Lisa Goldsmith—inf. diarh.—524-8750
3:15	Jody Albanese (Mike) laryn.—589-6151
3:30	Bonnie Secrist—589-4265
3:45	nose surgery
4:00	Mari Martin—Pap—522-5048
4:15	Mary Wadley—pain elbow—756-6346
4:30	Shelley Jones—stomach—756-6632

THURSDAY	
8:00	
8:15	
8:30	
8:45	
9:00	Rose Neptune—tetanus—526-3678
9:15	Tara Stimson (Roger) Pap—524-3107
9:30	Belinda Nelson—Bl. test—756-8032
9:45	Erin McKevitt (Ron) VDRL—589-3626
10:00	Cheryl Crupper—524-6505
10:15	physical
10:30	
10:45	
11:00	Cindy Hagedorn—756-7487
11:15	physical
11:30	Linda Clow (Mike)—589-4746
11:45	triplets—checkup
12:00	
12:15	(lunch)
12:30	
12:45	
1:00	Sandy Kirk—522-1190
1:15	physical
1:30	
1:45	
2:00	Kim Cantrell—all. shot—886-2108
2:15	Janet Pifer (Frederick)—529-5209
2:30	physical
2:45	
3:00	
3:15	Polly Troupe—BP—gastr.—886-4885
3:30	Cindy Taylor—OR—toenail—747-7501
3:45	
4:00	Ron Dillon—headaches—747-4858
4:15	Roger Daugherty—BP—524-1652
4:30	Brenda Kelser (Ron)—BP—589-5289

UNIT 23:4 COMPLETING MEDICAL RECORDS AND FORMS

1. statistical data sheets, medical history records
2. (Any 5 of the following) patient's name, address, telephone, marital status, gender, birthdate, place of employment, person responsible for account, insurance company, person referring
3. confidential, written consent, locked up
4. a. general data: name, address, age
   b. family history: diseases and conditions of patient's blood relatives; if family member dies, record cause of death and age at time of death
   c. past history: illnesses and treatments patient has had
   d. personal history: patient's marital and personal habits
   e. present illness: exact description of signs and symptoms patient is currently experiencing
5. a. S: single; b. M: married; c. W: widowed; d. D: divorced; e. O: negative or none; f. l&w: living and well; g. NA: not applicable; h. d: died

CHAPTER 23:5 COMPOSING BUSINESS LETTERS

1. a. collection: encourages patient to pay an account that is due
   b. appointment: informs patient of scheduled appointment
   c. recall: reminds patient to return for periodic examination
   d. consultation: requests another doctor to examine patient
   e. inquiry: seeks information
2. a. heading or letterhead, b. inside address, c. salutation, d. complimentary close, e. body, f. reference initials
3. a. 1st: state why letter is being written, b. 2nd: list main facts, c. 3rd: sign off or give final reminder
4. in block style all parts of letter are aligned at left margin; in modified block style heading, complimentary close and printed names begin at center with remainder of letter at left margin
5. date line, heading if letterhead is not present, complimentary close, keyed signature
6. a. Rose Toussaint, DDS; b. Dr. Toussaint
7. person dictating and person preparing the letter
8. a. OH, b. UT, c. AK, d. ID, e. WA, f. KY, g. MO, h. VA

CHAPTER 23:6 COMPLETING INSURANCE FORMS

1. statistical data, patient's information card, or in a computer database
2. the coverage may have changed
3. (Any 2 of the following) correct type of form, patient has completed any required parts, patient has signed forms in correct area, insured has signed forms if patient is a dependent
4. written release signed by patient and insured to provide information to insurance company; used when insurance forms are completed on computer and claims are filed electronically
5. insured
6. an all-purpose form required for any government-sponsored health care claims and accepted by all major insurance companies
7. International Classification of Diseases *Clinical Modifications (ICD-CM)*
8. identification of the disease or condition
9. in the order of importance
10. a. first three digits: single disease or group of closely related conditions
    b. fourth digit: makes disease more specific and tells location, cause, or stage of disease
    c. fifth digit: provides more specific information
11. bronchus
12. ICD-10-CM codes will be alphanumeric (letters and numbers) to accommodate more diseases and provide more specifics about a disease for tracking
13. *Physician's Current Procedural Terminology* (CPT)
14. five
15. further explain or change the meaning of a code
16. dash
17. letter, letters, NA, dash, all
18. Physician's National Provider number, ten-digit number inserted in box 24k and box 33 of HCFA-1500 form
19. "Signature on file," authorization to release information and assign benefits form must be completed
20. a. inpatient hospital, b. home, c. nursing home, d. outpatient hospital

CHAPTER 23:7 ASSIGNMENT SHEET #1 MAINTAINING A BOOKKEEPING SYSTEM

1. a. day sheet: daily record of all patients seen, charges incurred, and payments received
   b. statement-receipt: record of past balances, charges, payment received, current balance, and sometimes appointment date
   c. charge slip: charges for services rendered
   d. ledger card: total financial record

2. one copy can be mailed in place of or attached to an insurance form and thus eliminate the need for a separate insurance form
3. copies can be made and mailed to the patient
4. previous balance, charges, payment
5. a series of records are being recorded with one writing
6. line out neatly or void entire statement
7. received on account
8. amount charged by health care provider, negotiated or allowed amount according to the contract, amount the insurance company pays, amount of money the patient owes
9. a. an adjustment of $140 will be credited to the patient's account

   b. $48
10. (Any 4 of the following) name of patient, address, person responsible for account, family members in account, insurance information
11. preserve information in case of computer failure
12. $45

CHAPTER 23:7 ASSIGNMENT SHEET #2 MAINTAINING A BOOKKEEPING SYSTEM

			Chg.	Pay	CurB	PrevB	
5/1/—	Joan	Exam-PRO	149.00	50.00	99.00	00.00	John Smith
5/1/—	Mike	Endo	365.00	90.00	275.00	00.00	Mike Mendez
5/1/—	Mary	AM	165.00	——	264.00	99.00	John Smith
5/1/—	Jane	AR	145.00	95.00	325.00	275.00	Mike Mendez
5/1/—	Joe	EXT	325.00	100.00	489.00	264.00	John Smith
5/1/—	John	DENTURE	590.00	150.00	929.00	489.00	John Smith
5/1/—	John	ROA	——	540.00	389.00	929.00	John Smith

Total Deposit: 150.00 cash, 875.00 checks, 1,025.00 total

CHAPTER 23:7 ASSIGNMENT SHEET #3 MAINTAINING A BOOKKEEPING SYSTEM

			Chg	Pay	CurB	PrevB	
5/2/—	Jane	Exam-PRO	172.00	——	497.00	325.00	Mike Mendez
5/2/—	Mike	AM	213.00	85.00	625.00	497.00	Mike Mendez
5/2/—	Nellie	AR	148.00	210.00	563.00	625.00	Mike Mendez
5/2/—	Joe	DENTURE	1,825.00	850.00	1,904.00	929.00	John Smith
5/2/—	Mary	ENDO	297.00	125.00	2,076.00	1,904.00	John Smith
5/2/—	Brad	Exam	169.00	68.00	2,177.00	2,076.00	John Smith
5/2/—	Joe	ROA	——	1,956.38	220.62	2,177.00	John Smith
5/2/—	Mike	ROA	——	529.00	34.00	563.00	Mike Mendez

Total Deposit: 278.00 cash, 3,545.38 checks, 3,823.38 total

CHAPTER 23:8 ASSIGNMENT SHEET #1 WRITING CHECKS, DEPOSIT SLIPS, AND RECEIPTS

1. financial transactions
2. check, receipt
3. payee: person who receives payment

   originator or maker: person writing check or issuing payment

   endorsement: signature of the payee on the back of the check

4. so they cannot be altered or changed
5. (Any 4 of the following) correct amount, same amount on both lines, correct individual or agency as payee, accurate date, check signed by patient
6. prevents anyone from cashing the check if it is stolen
7. after the person takes it to the bank
8. receipt, proof, accurate, legible, ink
9. prevents loss or theft
10. $133.00, $1.18

CHAPTER 23:8 ASSIGNMENT SHEET #2 WRITING CHECKS, DEPOSIT SLIPS, AND RECEIPTS

Problems 1 and 2

No. 1 $ 802 $\frac{36}{100}$

Date 5/1/08

To ACE DRUG CO.

For PHARMACEUT.

Balance Brought Forward	19,102	39
Deposits		
Balance	19,102	39
Amount this check	802	36
Balance Carried Forward	18,300	03

Happy Doctor, MD
1 Healthy Lane
Fitness, OH 11133

No. 1

MAY 1 20 08

Pay to the Order of: ACE DRUG COMPANY $ 802 $\frac{36}{100}$

EIGHT HUNDRED TWO AND $\frac{36}{100}$ Dollars

First Money Bank
1 Rich Lane
Wealthy, OH 11133

Memo PHARMACEUTICALS By ____________

Problem 3

No. 2 $ 506 $\frac{28}{100}$

Date 5/2/08

To PHYSICIAN'S STATIONERY

For STATIONERY

Balance Brought Forward	18,300	03
Deposits		
Balance	18,300	03
Amount this check	506	28
Balance Carried Forward	17,793	75

Happy Doctor, MD
1 Healthy Lane
Fitness, OH 11133

No. 2

MAY 2 20 08

Pay to the Order of: PHYSICIAN'S STATIONERY SUPPLY COMPANY $ 506 $\frac{28}{100}$

FIVE HUNDRED SIX AND $\frac{28}{100}$ Dollars

First Money Bank
1 Rich Lane
Wealthy, OH 11133

Memo STATIONERY By ____________

Problem 4 (a–c)

4. a.

No. 1	No. 1	May 3 20 08
Date 5/3/08	Received From Mrs. James Johnson	
To Mrs. J. Johnson	One Thousand Five Hundred and 90/100	Dollars
For POA—Surgery	For Payment on account—surgery	
Amount 1,500 90/100 ck	$ 1,500 90/100 ck	*Student's Written Signature*

4. b.

No. 2	No. 2	May 3 20 08
Date 5/3/08	Received From Jerry Casper	
To Jerry Casper	One Thousand Two Hundred Fifty and 70/100 ———	Dollars
For ECG mach.	For ECG machine	
Amount $1,250 70/100 cash	$ 1,250 70/100 (cash)	*Student's Written Signature*

4. c.

No. 3	No. 3	May 3 20 08
Date 5/3/08	Received From Mrs. Kenneth Meyers	
To Mrs. Ken Meyers	Four Hundred Fifty and 10/100 ———	Dollars
For P.O.A.— bill	For Payment on account—medical bill	
Amount 450 10/100 ck.	$ 450 10/100 (ck.)	*Student's Written Signature*

Problem 5

Happy Doctor, MD
1 Healthy Lane
Fitness, OH 11133

Date May 3 20 08

Signature ____________
(If cash received)

First Money Bank
1 Rich Lane
Wealthy, OH 11133
0098-5567

Currency	1,250	00
Coin		70
Checks	1,500	90
	450	10
TOTAL	3,201	70
Less Cash	—	—
TOTAL DEPOSIT	3,201	70

Problem 6

No. 3	$ 3,225 00/100	
Date 5/3/08		
To BUSINESS RENTALS		
For OFFICE RENT		
Balance Brought Forward	17,793	75
Deposits	3,201	70
Balance	20,995	45
Amount this check	3,225	00
Balance Carried Forward	17,770	45

Happy Doctor, MD
1 Healthy Lane
Fitness, OH 11133

No. 3

MAY 3 20 08

Pay to the Order of: BUSINESS RENTALS, INC. $3,225 00/100

THREE THOUSAND TWO HUNDRED TWENTY FIVE AND 00/100 — Dollars

First Money Bank
1 Rich Lane
Wealthy, OH 11133

Memo OFFICE RENT By

Problem 7

No. 4	$ 478 85/100	
Date 5/4/08		
To TRI-COUNTY ELECTRIC		
For ELECTRIC BILL		
Balance Brought Forward	17,770	45
Deposits		
Balance	17,770	45
Amount this check	478	85
Balance Carried Forward	17,291	60

Happy Doctor, MD
1 Healthy Lane
Fitness, OH 11133

No. 4

MAY 4 20 08

Pay to the Order of: TRI-COUNTY ELECTRIC COMPANY $ 478 85/100

FOUR HUNDRED SEVENTY EIGHT AND 85/100 — Dollars

First Money Bank
1 Rich Lane
Wealthy, OH 11133

Memo ELECTRIC BILL By

Problem 8

No. 4
Date 5/5/08
To Mrs. Kathy Wrenner
For physical
Amount $250 00/100 ck.

No. 4 May 5 20 08

Received From Mrs. Kathy Wrenner

Two Hundred Fifty and 00/100 — Dollars

For Physical Exam

$ 250 00/100 (ck.) *Student's Written Signature*

Problem 9

Happy Doctor, MD
1 Healthy Lane
Fitness, OH 11133

Date May 5 20 08

Signature ____________
(If cash received)

First Money Bank
1 Rich Lane
Wealthy, OH 11133
0098-5567

Currency		
Coin		
Checks	250	00
TOTAL	250	00
Less Cash	–	–
TOTAL DEPOSIT	250	00

Problem 10

No. 5 $ 908 $\frac{10}{100}$
Date 5/6/08
To BOWMAN MEDICAL
For MED. SUPPLIES

Balance Brought Forward	17,291	60
Deposits	250	00
Balance	17,541	60
Amount this check	908	10
Balance Carried Forward	16,633	50

Happy Doctor, MD
1 Healthy Lane
Fitness, OH 11133

No. 5

MAY 6 20 08

Pay to the
Order of: BOWMAN MEDICAL SUPPLIES $ 908 $\frac{10}{100}$

NINE HUNDRED EIGHT AND $\frac{10}{100}$ Dollars

First Money Bank
1 Rich Lane
Wealthy, OH 11133

Memo MEDICAL SUPPLIES By ____________

Problem 11

No. 6 $ 604 $\frac{86}{100}$
Date 5/7/08
To CARDIO-SUPPLY
For EKG PAPERPADS

Balance Brought Forward	16,633	50
Deposits		
Balance	16,633	50
Amount this check	604	86
Balance Carried Forward	16,028	64

Happy Doctor, MD
1 Healthy Lane
Fitness, OH 11133

No. 6

MAY 7 20 08

Pay to the
Order of: CARDIO-SUPPLY COMPANY $ 604 $\frac{86}{100}$

SIX HUNDRED FOUR AND $\frac{86}{100}$ Dollars

First Money Bank
1 Rich Lane
Wealthy, OH 11133

Memo EKG PAPERPADS By ____________

CHAPTER 23:8 ASSIGNMENT SHEET #3 WRITING CHECKS, DEPOSIT SLIPS, AND RECEIPTS

Problems 1 and 2

No. 1 $ 10,220 00/100

Date 5/1/08

To J. JONES, M.D.

For X-RAY MACHINE

Balance Brought Forward	30,089	78
Deposits		
Balance	30,089	78
Amount this check	10,220	00
Balance Carried Forward	19,869	78

Happy Doctor, MD
1 Healthy Lane
Fitness, OH 11133

No. 1

MAY 1 20 08

Pay to the Order of: JEREMY JONES, M.D. $10,220 00/100

TEN THOUSAND TWO HUNDRED TWENTY AND 00/100 Dollars

First Money Bank
1 Rich Lane
Wealthy, OH 11133

Memo X-RAY MACHINE By

Problem 3

No. 2 $ 223 92/100

Date 5/1/08

To UNITED TELEPHONE

For TELEPHONE BILL

Balance Brought Forward	19,869	78
Deposits		
Balance	19,869	78
Amount this check	223	92
Balance Carried Forward	19,645	86

Happy Doctor, MD
1 Healthy Lane
Fitness, OH 11133

No. 2

MAY 1 20 08

Pay to the Order of: UNITED TELEPHONE COMPANY $ 223 92/100

TWO HUNDRED TWENTY THREE AND 92/100 Dollars

First Money Bank
1 Rich Lane
Wealthy, OH 11133

Memo TELEPHONE BILL By

Problem 4

No. 3 $ 1,102 30/100

Date 5/3/08

To MEDICO DG.

For DRUGS

Balance Brought Forward	19,645	86
Deposits		
Balance	19,645	86
Amount this check	1,102	30
Balance Carried Forward	18,543	56

Happy Doctor, MD
1 Healthy Lane
Fitness, OH 11133

No. 3

MAY 3 20 08

Pay to the Order of: MEDICO DRUG COMPANY $ 1,102 30/100

ONE THOUSAND ONE HUNDRED TWO AND 30/100 Dollars

First Money Bank
1 Rich Lane
Wealthy, OH 11133

Memo DRUGS By

Problem 5 (a–d)

5. a.

No. 1
Date 5/3/08
To Mrs. Estelle McCall
For ROA—surgery
Amount $1,206 55/100 ck.

No. 1 May 3 20 08
Received From Mrs. Estelle McCall
One Thousand Two Hundred Six and 55/100 —— Dollars
For Payment on account—surgery
$ 1,206 55/100 (ck.) *Student's Written Signature*

5. b.

No. 2
Date 5/3/08
To Mrs. Floyd Stark
For Physical
Amount $180 00/100 cash

No. 2 May 3 20 08
Received From Mrs. Floyd Stark
One Hundred Eighty and 00/100 —— Dollars
For Physical Exam
$ 180 00/100 (cash) *Student's Written Signature*

5. c

No. 3
Date 5/3/08
To Duane Yoder
For POA—suturing
Amount $225 00/100 ck.

No. 3 May 3 20 08
Received From Duane Yoder
Two Hundred Twenty Five and 00/100 —— Dollars
For Payment on account—suturing lacerations
$ 225 00/100 (cash) *Student's Written Signature*

5. d.

No. 4
Date 5/3/08
To Jim Johnson
For Fx. jaw
Amount $820 50/100 ck.

No. 4 May 3 20 08
Received From Jim Johnson
Eight Hundred Twenty and 50/100 —— Dollars
For Payment on account—fractured jaw
$ 820 50/100 (cash) *Student's Written Signature*

Problem 6

Happy Doctor, MD
1 Healthy Lane
Fitness, OH 11133

Date May 3 20 08

Signature ____________________
(If cash received)

First Money Bank
1 Rich Lane
Wealthy, OH 11133
0098-5567

Currency	180	00
Coin		
Checks	1,206	55
	225	00
	820	50
TOTAL	2,432	05
Less Cash	—	—
TOTAL DEPOSIT	2,432	05

Problem 7

No. 4 $ 4,200 75/100

Date 5/5/08

To BUSINESS RENTALS

For OFFICE RENT

Balance Brought Forward	18,543	56
Deposits	2,432	05
Balance	20,975	61
Amount this check	4,200	75
Balance Carried Forward	16,744	86

Happy Doctor, MD
1 Healthy Lane
Fitness, OH 11133

No. 4

MAY 5 20 08

Pay to the Order of: BUSINESS RENTALS $ 4,200 75/100

FOUR THOUSAND TWO HUNDRED AND 75/100 Dollars

First Money Bank
1 Rich Lane
Wealthy, OH 11133

Memo RENT By ____________________

Problem 8

No. 5	$ 52 $\frac{91}{100}$	
Date 5/6/08		
To MARIA SARDINA		
For OVERPAYMENT		
Balance Brought Forward	16,744	86
Deposits		
Balance	16,744	86
Amount this check	52	91
Balance Carried Forward	16,721	95

Happy Doctor, MD
1 Healthy Lane
Fitness, OH 11133

No. 5

MAY 6 20 08

Pay to the
Order of: MARIA SARDINA $ 52 $\frac{91}{100}$

FIFTY TWO AND $\frac{91}{100}$ Dollars

First Money Bank
1 Rich Lane
Wealthy, OH 11133

Memo OVERPAYMENT ON ACCOUNT By

Problem 9

No. 6	$ 3,929 $\frac{70}{100}$	
Date 5/7/08		
To GLOBAL INSURANCE		
For LIABILITY INS.		
Balance Brought Forward	16,721	95
Deposits		
Balance	16,721	95
Amount this check	3,929	70
Balance Carried Forward	12,792	25

Happy Doctor, MD
1 Healthy Lane
Fitness, OH 11133

No. 6

MAY 7 20 08

Pay to the
Order of: GLOBAL INSURANCE COMPANY $3,929 $\frac{70}{100}$

THREE THOUSAND NINE HUNDRED TWENTY NINE AND $\frac{70}{100}$ Dollars

First Money Bank
1 Rich Lane
Wealthy, OH 11133

Memo LIABILITY INSURANCE By

— NOTES —

— NOTES —

— NOTES —

— NOTES —

— NOTES —

— NOTES —

— NOTES —

— NOTES —

— NOTES —

— NOTES —

— NOTES —

— NOTES —

— NOTES —

— NOTES —

— NOTES —

— NOTES —

— NOTES —

— NOTES —

— NOTES —